DATE DUE

Understanding and Treating Violent Psychiatric Patients

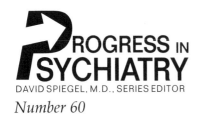

PROGRESS IN PSYCHIATRY

DAVID SPIEGEL, M.D., SERIES EDITOR

Number 60

Understanding and Treating Violent Psychiatric Patients

Edited by
Martha L. Crowner, M.D.

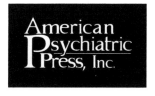

American
Psychiatric
Press, Inc.

Washington, DC
London, England

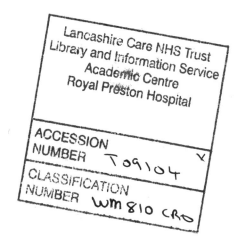

Copyright © 2000 American Psychiatric Press, Inc.

ALL RIGHTS RESERVED
Manufactured in the United States of America on acid-free paper
03 02 01 00   4 3 2 1
First Edition

American Psychiatric Press, Inc.
1400 K Street, N.W., Washington, DC 20005
www.appi.org

Library of Congress Cataloging-in-Publication Data
Understanding and treating violent psychiatric patients /   edited by Martha L. Crowner.—1st ed.
p. cm. — (Progress in psychiatry ; #60)
Includes bibliographical references and index.
ISBN 0-88048-752-6
1. Psychiatric hospital care. 2. Violence in psychiatric hospitals. 3. Psychiatric hospital patients. I. Crowner, Martha, 1956– II. Progress in psychiatry series ; #60.

RC439.4 .U536 2000
362.2′1—dc21

99-049869

British Library Cataloguing in Publication Data
A CIP record is available from the British Library.

Contents

Section II
Approaches to Understanding
Violent Patients

Contributors

Niels C. Beck, Ph.D.
Professor, Department of Psychiatry and Neurology, University of Missouri—Columbia, Columbia, Missouri

Laura Jane Bernay, M.D.
Clinical Assistant Professor of Psychiatry, New York University School of Medicine, New York, New York

Patrick W. Corrigan, Psy.D.
Executive Director, University of Chicago Center for Psychiatric Rehabilitation, Tinley Park, Illinois; Associate Professor of Psychiatry, University of Chicago, Chicago, Illinois

Martha L. Crowner, M.D.
Manhattan Psychiatric Center, Ward's Island, New York; Clinical Associate Professor of Psychiatry, New York University School of Medicine, New York, New York

Devitt J. Elverson, M.D.
Director, Inpatient Psychiatry and Associate Vice-Chairman of Psychiatry, Coney Island Hospital, Brooklyn, New York; Clinical Associate Professor of Psychiatry, State University of New York Health Science Center at Brooklyn, New York

Menahem Krakowski, M.D., Ph.D.
Research Psychiatrist, Nathan Kline Institute for Psychiatric Research, Orangeburg, New York; Assistant Professor of Psychiatry, New York University School of Medicine, New York, New York

Richard P. Malone, M.D.
Associate Professor of Psychiatry, Department of Psychiatry, and Director, Child and Adolescent Psychiatry Research, MCP Hahnemann University School of Medicine, Philadelphia, Pennsylvania

Anthony A. Menditto, Ph.D.
Director, Psychosocial Rehabilitation Services, Fulton State Hospital; Clinical Assistant Professor, Department of Psychiatry and Neurology, University of Missouri—Columbia, Columbia, Missouri

John Monahan, Ph.D.
Henry and Grace Doherty Professor of Law and Professor of Psychology and Legal Medicine, University of Virginia School of Law, Charlottesville, Virginia

Kim T. Mueser, Ph.D.
Professor, New Hampshire–Dartmouth Psychiatric Research Center, Concord, New Hampshire

A. Jonathan Porteus, M.A.
Director of Research and Evaluation, Daytop Village, Inc., New York, New York; Director, Trauma and Addiction Services, The New York Center for Neuropsychology and Forensic Behavioral Science, Brooklyn, New York

Paul Stuve, Ph.D.
Program Coordinator, Fulton State Hospital; Clinical Assistant Professor, Department of Psychiatry and Neurology, University of Missouri—Columbia, Columbia, Missouri

Zebulon Taintor, M.D.
Professor and Vice Chairman, Department of Psychiatry, New York University Medical Center, New York, New York

Introduction to the Progress in Psychiatry Series

The Progress in Psychiatry Series is designed to capture in print the excitement that comes from assembling a diverse group of experts from various locations to examine in detail the newest information about a developing aspect of psychiatry. This series emerged as a collaboration between the American Psychiatric Association's (APA) Scientific Program Committee and the American Psychiatric Press, Inc. Great interest is generated by a number of the symposia presented each year at the APA annual meeting, and we realized that much of the information presented there, carefully assembled by people who are deeply immersed in a given area, would unfortunately not appear together in print. The symposia sessions at the annual meetings provide an unusual opportunity for experts who otherwise might not meet on the same platform to share their diverse viewpoints for a period of 3 hours. Some new themes are repeatedly reinforced and gain credence, whereas in other instances disagreements emerge, enabling the audience and now the reader to reach informed decisions about new directions in the field. The Progress in Psychiatry Series allows us to publish and capture some of the best of the symposia and thus provide an in-depth treatment of specific areas that might not otherwise be presented in broader review formats.

Psychiatry is, by nature, an interface discipline, combining the study of mind and brain, of individual and social environments, of the humane and the scientific. Therefore, progress in the field is rarely linear—it often comes from unexpected sources. Furthermore, new developments emerge from an array of viewpoints that do not necessarily provide immediate agreement but rather expert examination of the issues. We intend to present innovative ideas and data that will enable the reader to participate in this process.

We believe the Progress in Psychiatry Series will provide you with an opportunity to review timely, new information in specific fields of interest as they are developing. We hope you find that the excitement of the presentations is captured in the written word and that this book proves to be informative and enjoyable reading.

David Spiegel, M.D.
Series Editor
Progress in Psychiatry Series

Introduction

Violent patients readily provoke fear, anger, and revulsion. In response, clinicians tend to keep their distance. They avoid getting to know the patient as a complex person with an illness, but only discern behavior that must be controlled. They may then accomplish management of violence, but they fail to analyze or understand it in a broader context. Treatment also suffers. Violent patients are too often contained and controlled while treatment is a distant priority and second rate compared with that offered to nonviolent patients.

Wider, societal forces, intent on community safety and quality of life, also press for containment of individuals who are violent or threatening or have been in the past. Although the clinician may be most at ease serving solely the patient's interests—autonomy, alleviation of suffering, and lessening of disability—a violent patient creates obligations to both community and individual interests, which often conflict.

This book's title, *Understanding and Treating Violent Psychiatric Patients,* was chosen to underscore the mental health profession's obligation to these patients. We are compelled to extend our goals beyond containment and behavioral control to understanding, to complete assessment and accurate diagnosis, and to humane and effective treatment. I have sorted this volume's chapters into two groups. The first group are practical guides to assessment, management, and treatment, while the second group of chapters are more conceptual and more broadly focused approaches to understanding.

The first section consists of five chapters. In Chapter 1, I present clinical advice based not only on experience but also on data from clinical trials. I discuss how violence presents in different diagnostic groups, review common treatment problems among violent adult inpatients, and provide a brief guide to long-term pharmacological treatments.

Dr. Malone's chapter (Chapter 2) is the only one in this book to consider children and adolescents. The assessments Dr. Malone describes are observational scales and self-report, interview, and laboratory measures. He also reviews and evaluates the existing literature on controlled trials of medications in children and adolescents with aggression related to disruptive disorders, primarily conduct disorder, but sometimes attention-deficit/hyperactivity disorder.

In Chapter 3, Drs. Bernay and Elverson review the use of verbal techniques, isolation or quiet room, pharmacological measures, and restraint and seclusion. Their discussion of medication choices is extensive and specific, but their discussion of restraint and seclusion is still more extensive.

Chapter 4, by Drs. Corrigan and Mueser, can serve as an overview of a variety of behavioral approaches—approaches that should be more familar to psychiatrists. The methods the authors outline—behavioral family therapy, social skills training, and cognitive skills training—attempt to ameliorate patient limitations that can contribute to violent behavior. These include their vulnerability to overarousal, cognitive deficits, and lack of social support. Drs. Corrigan and Mueser also describe behavioral strategies to de-escalate aggression, such as social extinction and contingent observation.

In Chapter 5, Dr. Menditto and his colleagues give a detailed account of a token economy, a topic treated only briefly by Drs. Corrigan and Mueser in Chapter 4. The token economy, modeled after that created by Paul and Lentz,[1] has been functioning for several years at Fulton State Hospital in Missouri. It is a comprehensive treatment program that has a demonstrated ability to increase adaptive behavior and decrease maladaptive behavior such as assault.

The four chapters in the second section are different conceptual approaches to understanding violent behavior in widely different contexts. In Chapter 6, I describe a study of assaults between psychiatric inpatients that used a system of video cameras installed in each corner of a dayroom on a ward of a large state psychiatric hospital. In Chapter 7, Mr. Porteus and Dr. Taintor explore the relationship between dissociation and violence, a topic of great public interest that is often sensationalized but subject to little serious study. Dr. Krakowski, in Chapter 8, discusses the origins of impulse control. He also provides a thoughtful review of the data on impulsivity and serotonergic dysfunction. He then integrates both topics as he considers the clinical presentation of impulsive patients, particularly those with borderline and antisocial personality disorders. In the final chapter, Dr. Monahan reviews current thinking on the relationship between psychiatric disorder and violence in the general population.

I hope this volume helps clinicians meet these especially challenging patients with greater curiosity, if not understanding, and with a systematic approach to assessment and humane and effective treatment.

Martha L. Crowner, M.D.

---

[1] Paul GL, Lentz RJ: *Psychosocial Treatment of Chronic Mental Patients: Milieu Versus Social-Learning Programs.* Cambridge, MA, Harvard University Press, 1977.

SECTION I

Treatment Strategies for Violent Patients

CHAPTER 1

A Brief Guide to the Assessment and Pharmacological Treatment of Violent Adult Psychiatric Inpatients

Martha L. Crowner, M.D.

After a serious assault, the entire ward, staff and patients, is in an uproar. Staff are often beside themselves—exasperated, angry, and terrified. The patient is usually humiliated, angry, and fearful. An assault imposes extraordinary challenges to the treating psychiatrist: above all, to remain rational and systematic, but also to understand what happened, devise a treatment plan, and lead others. The psychiatrist should not rush into a "one size fits all" plan, but remember that he or she is charged with treating a violent patient, not violence. Patients can become violent for very different reasons, just as they stop in response to different treatments.

In this chapter I review the investigation of violent incidents at inpatient facilities, the assessment of violent patients, and, finally, the patients' long-term treatment. Drs. Bernay and Elverson review emergency containment of dangerous patients in another chapter in this volume (see Chapter 3). In this chapter my discussion of treatments concentrates on pharmacological treatments, but I do not mean to imply that these are sufficient. Other chapters in this volume outline psychosocial treatments (see Chapters 4 and 5). Assessment and treatment of violent patients have been reviewed at length elsewhere, by Tardiff (1996) and Volavka (1995). This chapter is intended to be much less comprehensive, offering a general clinical approach with selected references. I review treatment problems most common in violent inpatients, particularly severely and chronically ill patients. The chapter draws on my clinical and research experience on the secure care unit of a large

New York State inpatient facility, the clinical expertise of Dr. Brian Anderson, and the work of Drs. Menahem Krakowski and Jan Volavka.

Assessment of Violent Incidents and Violent Inpatients

Initial Approach

After the immediate safety of patient and staff has been assured, a violent incident demands a thorough investigation and case review. The best person for this job is often a consulting psychiatrist, someone who can provide a fresh, hopeful approach.

The initial assessment may be separated into three parts: an interview with the patient-assailant, an interview with staff and victim, and a review of the patient's records.

The initial patient interview might be impossible or very brief, so the consultant should try to collect as much information as possible from other sources in order to develop hypotheses that can be tested when the patient is more accessible. Patients will usually press to relate their version of events. Sooner or later, they should be heard out. Assailant interviews can help the patient save face and can help the psychiatrist develop an empathic working relationship with the patient.

Private, individual interviews with the victim, the nurse on duty, other staff members, and sometimes other patients can often provide more accurate and more detailed factual information than written records. These interviews can also elicit crucial subjective information that can guide management decisions—for instance, how staff members feel about what happened and how apprehensive they are about working with the patient in the future. The interviews serve another important function in that they communicate personal concern and demonstrate quick, effective action.

The goals of the investigation of the incident are to understand what happened in the assault and before. This can lead to an appreciation of assailant motivation and psychopathology and, naturally, to rational treatment planning. The goals of the patient case review are to learn the course of assaultiveness, both in and out of the hospital, and to determine how assaultiveness may be related to psychopathology. If the assault is related to decompensation, a deterioration in functioning and psychopathology, the investigating psychiatrist should discover its possible causes.

The Assault and Its Antecedents

All aggressive behavior between patients is not equivalent; it can range from a slap, push, or shove, perhaps in play or irritation, to serious attempts to hurt (Crowner et al. 1994). It is important to learn exactly what the assailant did. The degree of the assault's seriousness or potential seriousness is most significant in deciding how much containment and supervision the patient requires. The seriousness can be gauged by learning where the blows landed, if a weapon of any type was used, what injuries resulted, and how staff intervened. Many assaults could have been more injurious if staff had not intervened. Some injuries are so severe that they prompt the victim or the hospital administration to consider pressing legal charges (Volavka et al. 1995a).

The consultant should learn about the relationship between victim and assailant and what happened between them just before the assault. There may have been physical contact or proximity; perhaps the victim jostled the assailant while standing in line or the victim may have been an employee helping an incapacitated patient dress or groom. There could have been words between the assailant and victim before the assault: an argument, threats, or insults. Perhaps a staff member denied a request or tried to set limits. Patients' recounting of what happened and why they did what they did can suggest an interaction between victim and assailant that the assailant misinterpreted or reacted to with disproportionate anger (Crowner et al. 1995). In this way, the investigation can further an understanding of the assailant's psychopathology and motivation.

Violence and Psychopathology, or How and Why Patients Become Assaultive

The following examples demonstrate ways in which interpersonal interactions, victim psychopathology, and assailant psychopathology can precipitate assault.

Coercion

Aggression in humans can be classified, following a well-accepted but very simple classification system, as instrumental/predatory or explosive/affective (Eichelman 1990). For example, one patient obtains valuables or sexual gratification from another through threats, assault, or theft. The second patient then assaults the first in self-defense or retaliation. The first patient's behavior illustrates *predatory,* or instrumental, aggression—aggression motivated primarily by a desire for some tangible thing, privileges, or control. An example of explosive/affective aggression occurs when a patient becomes enraged and tries to throttle another patient who has been tying up the telephone. Aggression may be both instrumental and explosive. For example, the enraged patient's aggression has intended or unintended instrumental results as the talkative patient becomes more likely to give up the telephone.

Psychosis

Psychotic patients may be disorganized or have prominent, systematized delusional systems. In patients with organized delusions, violence is more often directed at a specific person, perhaps the center of the delusional system, a person seen as persecuting or depriving the patient in some way. The target of these patients is often a friend or family member, so the assaults are committed by patients outside the hospital (Krakowski et al. 1986). In a community sample, paranoid delusions and delusions of mind control and thought insertion were associated with violence (Link and Stueve 1994).

In disorganized psychotic patients, violence is less focused, less planned, and often less dangerous (Krakowski et al. 1986). More disorganized paranoid patients may interpret a bump or shove, or physical closeness, as an intrusion or a homosexual threat. Command hallucinations have been related to serious crimes in the community (Hafner and Boker 1982) and can also precipitate assaults in psychiatric hospitals.

Mania

Patients in a manic episode have been described as more angry and agitated than assaultive (Krakowski et al. 1986), but they can become assaultive toward staff when they are contained, restricted, or pressed to comply. Containment and routine are the norm in any institution, so staff members often struggle with these patients. Because they are so irritable, they often overreact to intrusions, shouts, or insults from other patients. Because they are loud, overly active, intrusive, and belligerent, they provoke other patients. Although another patient may throw the first blow, the manic patient can retaliate and become identified as the aggressor.

Dementia in the Elderly

Aggression in elderly patients with dementia is usually reactive and unplanned. Bridges-Parlet et al. (1994) studied the precipitants of physical aggression in 20 elderly nursing home residents with dementia, most with severe dementia. Of the 20 subjects, 13 were women and 10 were men. The mean age of the residents was 77 years, with a range from 65 to 95. The investigators found that only 5 of 28 assaults detected (18%) were directed toward other residents, often as a result of "uninvited advances," such as lying in the assailant's bed. Twenty-three assaults were directed toward staff. Twenty of these (87%) occurred when staff were bathing, toileting, grooming, dressing, or redirecting. Only 13% of the aggressive episodes toward staff had no identifiable precipitant.

Temporal Lobe Epilepsy

The relationship between seizure disorders, particularly temporal lobe epilepsy, and violence has been addressed elegantly and in depth by Dr. Volavka (1995). He summarized his discussion in this way: "[T]he aggressive behavior that may occasionally occur during and immediately after psychomotor seizures is usually trivial, appears purposeless, may reflect confusion, and is probably increased or even induced by attempts to restrain the patient" (p. 103). As in other groups, violence in patients with temporal lobe epilepsy is often reactive. When a patient is in the midst of a seizure, staff members should remain watchful and direct the patient away from others, but keep a distance.

Head Trauma

Patients who have suffered head trauma are a nonrandom sample. Certain characteristics, such as risk taking and substance abuse, make serious accidents—and a tendency to be violent—more likely. This is probably less true of the victims of military combat. For this reason, the study of Grafman et al. (1996) is particularly useful in understanding the relationship between violence and head trauma.

Grafman et al. studied 279 Vietnam veterans who had sustained penetrating head injuries in service and 57 control subjects matched for age, education, and service in Vietnam. Aggression was broadly defined to include verbal aggression, irritability, and physical fights and rated by family members. As a whole, the group with head injury exhibited more aggression than the control group. Patients with frontal ventromedial lesions were more aggressive than patients with lesions in other areas. Frontal lobe dysfunction may impair patients' abilities to interact in social situations. Rather than restraining themselves, they tend to react quickly and aggressively to immediate provocations (Lau and Pihl 1995).

Course of Assaultiveness and Course of the Illness

Typically, the prevalence of assault is greatest in the first few weeks following admission, after which its frequency declines steeply and levels off (Volavka 1995, p. 252). This pattern can be explained in several ways. Assaultiveness soon after admission can be related to substance abuse in the community (Myers and Dunner 1984). Acute psychosis and untreated mania, which are common reasons for admission, are associated with an increased risk of assaultiveness (Krakowski et al. 1986). Because the majority of a group of patients tend to respond to treatment, the prevalence of assaultiveness in a group tends to decline after treatment is instituted.

When patients are assaultive after their initial few weeks of hospitalization, the behavior may or may not be related to psychopathology. The assault may be an indication of psychopathology that has continuously resisted treatment or of pathology that, while initially responsive, has recurred. Some patients are intermittently but consistently violent, typically patients whose psychopathology is difficult to treat, such as those with personality disorders so severe they require hospitalization or those with treatment-refractory schizophrenia. For other patients, there may have been a point at which their functioning and psychopathology began to deteriorate, followed by assaultiveness. It is also important to remember that assaults are not always clearly related to assailant psychopathology. At times, patients react to external, interpersonal stressors, such as bullying and threats or intimidation.

If the assailant has had a relapse, it is important to learn when it started and with what it was associated. The reemergence of psychosis may be associated with an increased risk of assaultive behavior, and the severity of psychotic symptoms can be reflected in the frequency of violent incidents (Krakowski et al. 1986). The violent event and overall functional decline may be related to many possible factors. Among those to consider are acute external stressors, such as losses, disappointments, conflicts with family, a change in ward, a recent home pass, and learning of an HIV diagnosis. Surreptitious illegal drug use can also cause an acute change in behavior and symptoms, so a urine toxicology screen is indicated. General medical problems may also cause behavioral changes. For example, patients may become confused and agitated when they are hypoglycemic or suffer an acute febrile illness.

Noncompliance with prescribed drugs is a frequent precipitant of decompensation. The consultant should ask the ward nurse if the patient has been taking prescribed medication and closely inspect the nurses' medication record. Patients sometimes pretend to swallow their tablets but toss them in a trashcan or deposit them in their pockets, in bedside drawers, under the mattress, in a dark corner, and so forth. A thorough tablet search can uncover this cause for decompensation.

History of Violence, or Assaultiveness Outside the Hospital

A review of the patient's more distant history may reveal evidence of prior violent behavior. A history of violence can predict similar behavior on the ward and after discharge. The circumstances or context of past violence—for example, medication noncompliance or illegal drug abuse—may predict the circumstances of more recent violence. Beyond assaults in hospitals, the psychiatrist should review records for reports of violent crime, assaults against family members (which often do not result in criminal charges but do result in psychiatric admissions), violent suicide attempts, and substance abuse.

Arrests and convictions for violent, but not nonviolent, crime distinguished a group of 77 violent state hospital inpatients from a group of 40 nonviolent ones, a significant difference ($P < 0.05$). The violent patients were also more likely than the nonviolent patients to have made violent suicide attempts, but the difference was a trend and not statistically significant ($P = 0.08$). A history of nonviolent suicide attempts, such as superficial cutting and overdosing, did not distinguish the groups (Convit et al. 1988). The violent group of inpatients were consecutive admissions to the Intensive Psychiatric Service at the Manhattan Psychiatric Center (see Chapter 6, this volume); the nonviolent patients had been on other wards for at least 6 months, where they had never been seriously violent. The distributions of the variables age, chronicity of illness, gender, and race for the two groups were matched as closely as possible. The mean age was approximately 32 years for both groups, with a mean duration of illness of 12–14 years. Seventy percent of the violent sample and 80% of the control sample were male. Eighty-eight percent of the violent sample were nonwhite, as were 77% of the control sample, which reflected the composition of the entire hospital population. Seventy-nine percent of the violent group and 85% of the control group were diagnosed with schizophrenia by a consensus of two psychiatrists on the basis of DSM-III criteria (American Psychiatric Association 1980).

Treatment of Violent Inpatients

Approach to Treatment

The preceding discussion emphasized the need for thorough assessment and careful diagnosis. Violence itself is only a behavior, which may be associated with many types of psychopathology. The psychiatrist may elect to treat a syndrome (e.g., schizophrenia) or the symptoms associated with violence (e.g., impulsivity, hostility, paranoia, or agitation). The safest, most parsimonious approach is to identify and aggressively treat a syndrome, or, in other words, to use the smallest number of drugs for the largest number of symptoms. This is easier done when there are well-established treatments for the patient's diagnosis, as is the case for schizophrenia or bipolar disorder. For other conditions, such as borderline personality disorder or the sequelae of head trauma, treatment is necessarily more symptomatic.

For an example of unsuccessful symptomatic treatment, consider the case of a chronically psychotic patient with restlessness, frequent screaming, and intrusiveness who was treated with a typical neuroleptic, benzodiazepines for agitation, and beta-blockers for aggressivity. The patient's underlying condition, which could have been treatment-resistant schizophrenia or mania with psychotic symptoms or schizoaffective disorder, was not adequately identified or treated. A more parsimonious and effective strategy would have been to use mood stabilizers or an atypical neuroleptic. Here, purely symptomatic treatment was a poor substitute for adequate treatment of the patient's illness.

This case illustrates several treatment points. Benzodiazepines may be effective temporarily, but with long-term use patients develop tolerance and dependence. Disinhibition of aggressive impulses has been reported with benzodiazepines, but it appears to be quite rare (Dietch and Jennings 1988). The patient in the example could have an affective disorder with a particularly malignant course. Over 40% of current-day patients with bipolar disorder have recurrent affective syndromes, associated with poorer longitudinal courses (Goldberg et al. 1995). Such a diagnosis should be considered for chronically ill patients who have not responded adequately to neuroleptics alone; who are often agitated, very active, intrusive, and provocative; and who have trouble conforming to ward expectations.

Early steps in planning of pharmacological treatment are assessment of compliance and side effects. In this section I begin with a short discussion of compliance and of the association of akathisia and violence. After considering the difficulties and limitations of treatment studies, I review the literature on treatment with beta-blockers, lithium, and carbamazepine. The effectiveness of atypical neuroleptics for hostility in schizophrenia, and the treatment of impulsivity and hostility with selective serotonin reuptake inhibitors (SSRIs), are then addressed.

Compliance

Treatment noncompliance cuts across diagnostic boundaries. It is a frequent cause of relapse in patients with schizophrenia, schizoaffective disorder, or bipolar disorder. Compliance and a related concept, insight, have been the object of much recent academic interest. Compliance may be related to insight, to attitudes to treatment (including delusions about treatment), to side effects and beneficial effects, and to the relationship between physician and patient (Kemp and David 1996). Some aspects of insight may be related to some neuropsychological variables, but the relationship between compliance and global cognitive ability is not strong.

Compliance can improve through psychosocial interventions, as exemplified by the compliance therapy for psychotic patients of Kemp and colleagues (1996). In 4–6 sessions of 20–60 minutes' duration, the clinician reviews the symptoms of the illness and the risks and benefits of treatment, explores the ambivalence and the stigma of taking drugs, and presents drugs as a means of relapse prevention. Compliance can improve if psychiatrists vigorously treat adverse effects. They should strive to discover the most acceptable route, number of doses, and timing of doses for each individual patient. Compliance may improve with decanoate or concentrate preparations.

When patients with schizophrenia are violent and refuse oral medications, the treating psychiatrist has a strong case for requesting treatment over objection, either decanoate preparations or electroconvulsive therapy. With neuroleptic treatment, insight tends to improve, along with other psychopathological and cognitive variables, so patients may willingly accept treatment that was initially forced.

Akathisia and Violence

Akathisia is a neuroleptic side effect with prevalence commonly estimated at 20%, with greater prevalence in patients on higher-potency agents (Ayd 1961). Most investigators agree that akathisia has both a motor and a subjective component. The subjective component has been described as a sense of inner restlessness or agitation or dysphoria that can be intense. The distress may lead to worsened symptoms of anxiety, depression, and psychosis (Van Putten et al. 1974). In anecdotal reports, the subjective component of akathisia has been associated with suicidal or homicidal ideas or acts (Drake and Ehrlich 1985; Shear et al. 1983). Keckich (1978) and Schulte (1985) reported on patients whose assaultiveness was apparently associated with akathisia. Herrera et al. (1988) reported significantly more violent episodes among a group of schizophrenic inpatients during a 6-week haloperidol trial than during crossover trials of either placebo or low-potency drugs (chlorpromazine or clozapine). Akathisia was suggested as a possible cause of the increased violence.

Limitations of Treatment Studies

Some of the limitations of reports of studies of treatments for aggression are similar to those of other treatment studies; others are peculiar to studies of treatments for aggression. As with reports of treatments for other conditions, reports of treatments for violent patients are often anecdotal, retrospective, or open; when prospective experimental trials are available, the sample sizes are small or without placebo control groups. Some investigators study diagnostically mixed groups of patients, an approach that makes results difficult to interpret. Consideration of pharmacokinetic interactions or indirect mechanisms of action (e.g., treatment of akathisia) is often inadequate. As in other treatment reports, there is a reporting bias, in that ineffective trials are not reported.

Treatment studies for aggression have unique difficulties. Violence is usually a rare event, so investigators need a long baseline period and a long treatment phase to see a significant effect. In case reports it often happens that patients are started on experimental treatments soon after a violent incident, when clinicians are most motivated. Because violence is rare, patients are likely be less violent in the future, so any treatment might seem effective. To circumvent the problem of a rare dependent variable (i.e., violence), investigators might choose another variable, such as hostility or impulsivity, a dependent variable that may be more fundamental than violent behavior.

Medications in Long-Term Treatment of Aggression

Beta-Blockers

Most experience with beta-blockers for the treatment of aggression has been with patients with organic brain disease or injury. In the only well-controlled study—a double-blind, placebo-controlled, crossover trial of propranolol for assaultive behavior in patients with dementia (Green-dyke et al. 1986)—7 of 9 subjects had a positive response to the propranolol in that their assaultive behavior decreased. In a second double-blind, placebo-controlled study (Ratey et al. 1992), the experimental groups differed in baseline aggression, so the results are difficult to interpret.

When patients with schizophrenia are treated with beta-blockers (Sheppard 1979; Sorgi et al. 1986), possible pharmacokinetic interactions with neuroleptics must be considered. Propranolol is known to raise blood levels of chlorpromazine and thioridazine (Miller and Rampling 1982; Vestral et al. 1979). It may also be that propranolol is indirectly treating aggression in these patient by treating akathisia, because its efficacy for this indication is well documented (Adler et al. 1988; Lipinski et al. 1984).

Lithium and Carbamazepine

Lithium has been used in groups of offenders with antisocial and other personality disorders (Sheard 1971, 1975) and chronic psychotic patients (Martorano 1972). In this volume (see Chapter 2) Dr. Malone reviews the use of lithium in the treatment of aggressive children and adolescents. Sheard (1984) concluded that lithium was effective across diagnostic groups. It was particularly effective in patients in whom anger, rage, and irritability were prominent and easily triggered. When psychotic patients are treated with lithium, the questions of neuroleptic-lithium interactions and diagnostic uncertainty arise (Van Putten and Sanders 1975). Lithium may increase intracellular levels of neuroleptics (Nemes et al. 1986).

Similar issues are pertinent to a consideration of the literature on the use of carbamazepine in the treatment of aggression. Placebo-controlled studies of carbamazepine are few and show negative results (Sheard 1984).

Clozapine and Risperidone

A growing literature has documented the efficacy of clozapine in decreasing hostility and aggression in patients with schizophrenia. This efficacy could be attributed to clozapine's superior ability to treat positive symptoms in patients with treatment-resistant schizophrenia, but the effect has been shown to be above and beyond clozapine's effect on positive symptoms. There is much less literature on risperidone, but one study suggests it has effects similar to those of clozapine.

Wilson (1992) reviewed the hospital charts of the first 37 patients at a state psychiatric hospital to start treatment with clozapine. Over the 6-month review period, the 37 patients were involved in fewer and fewer violent incidents. Ratey et al. (1993) completed a retrospective chart review for 5 patients taking clozapine and found that "although psychotic symptoms were not greatly affected by the drug, the overall frequency of assaults, self-abuse, and the use of seclusion, mechanical restraint, and chemical restraint was reduced in the subjects" (p. 219).

Chiles et al. (1994) compared the frequency of episodes of seclusion and restraint 12 weeks before clozapine treatment and 12 weeks after among 115 chronic state hospital patients. Nurses' Observation Scale for Inpatient Evaluation (NOSIE; Guy 1976, p. 271) ratings were obtained for 84 of this group. The frequency of seclusion and restraint declined significantly. Improvement on all NOSIE subscales except physical retardation was noted. Volavka et al. (1995b) studied Brief Psychiatric Rating Scale (BPRS; Guy 1976, p. 157) scores in records of 223 New York State inpatients, comparing change in hostility item to change in psychosis factor. They hypothesized that clozapine would result in a change in hostility that would be not associated with a change in psychosis (i.e., the change still remained significant after accounting for the change in psychosis). Post hoc regression analyses revealed a significant improvement in hostility after the improvement in psychosis was accounted for.

Chengappa and colleagues (1999) found that clozapine is also useful in treating severely ill patients with borderline personality disorder and persistent psychosis. They compared equal time periods, before and after clozapine treatment, for seven subjects, all white women in state psychiatric hospitals. With clozapine, incidents of self-mutilation and injuries to others decreased significantly.

Czobor and colleagues (1995) found similar results for risperidone. They examined psychopathology scores from 139 patients enrolled in a

9-week multicenter placebo-controlled, double-blind study of the effects of risperidone. The investigators took as their dependent variable change in hostility, and as a covariate change in psychosis, in order to test for a selective effect (i.e., a change in hostility unrelated to change in psychosis). They found that risperidone had a greater selective effect on hostility than did either haloperidol or placebo.

Selective Serotonin Reuptake Inhibitors

Fluoxetine has been used with patients with personality disorders in small, open-label trials for the treatment of aggressive, impulsive behavior, as well as many other symptoms (Coccaro et al. 1989, 1990; Cornelius et al. 1990; Markovitz et al. 1991). There is also a case report of the treatment of severe agitation and assaultiveness in a 48-year-old man with dementia secondary to trauma (Sobin et al. 1989). Coccaro et al. (1990) openly treated patients with borderline or antisocial personality disorders for 6 weeks with escalating doses of fluoxetine up to 60 mg/day. Weekly ratings of assault decreased in 2 of 3 patients. Markovitz et al. (1991) treated 22 patients with borderline or schizotypal personality disorders in a 12-week trial at doses increasing to 80 mg/day. Patients showed significant decreases in self-mutilation and other affective and psychotic symptoms, as measured by responses to self-assessment questionnaires. Cornelius et al. (1990) openly treated 5 patients with borderline personality disorder with 20–40 mg/day for 8 weeks, with resulting decreases in measures of impulsivity, depression, and suicidality, but not in hostility.

Summary

Assault by patients is rare, so many clinicians are often at a loss when confronted by a serious incident on an inpatient ward. In this chapter I have provided a clinician's quick guide to how to complete an assessment of the incident and the patient and then how to direct subsequent treatment. I have outlined a course of thinking about the assault itself and the interpersonal interaction before it occurs with examples of how and why patients from different diagnostic groups typically assault. I discussed how violence may be related to decompensation. I also discussed how violence in the patient's history may predict the circumstances of more recent events. The chapter concluded with a short review of pharmacological treatments for long-term, not emergency, treatment of violent patients, including beta-blockers, lithium, carbamazepine, clozapine, risperidone, and SSRIs.

Clinicians treat violent patients, not violence. It follows that each assault must be understood in the context of a particular patient in a particular situation. To prevent further incidents, it is important to learn the purpose or meaning of the assault for the patient as well as how it may result from circumstances and psychopathology. Patients with many different pathologies become violent and require many different treatments.

References

Adler LA, Reiter S, Corwin J, et al: Neuroleptic-induced akathisia: propranolol versus benztropine (letter). J Biol Psychiatry 23:211–213, 1988

American Psychiatric Association: Diagnostic and Statistical Manual of Mental Disorders, 3rd Edition. Washington, DC, American Psychiatric Association, 1980

Ayd FJ: A survey of drug-induced extrapyramidal reactions. JAMA 175:1054–1060, 1961

Bridges-Parlet S, Knopman D, Thompson T: A descriptive study of physically aggressive behavior in dementia by direct observation. J Am Geriatr Soc 42:192–197, 1994

Chengappa KN, Egeling T, Kang JS, et al: Clozapine reduces severe self-mutilation and aggression in psychotic patients with borderline personality disorder. J Clin Psychiatry 60:477–484, 1999

Chiles JA, Davidson P, McBride D: Effects of clozapine on use of seclusion and restraint at a state hospital. Hospital and Community Psychiatry 45:269–271, 1994

Coccaro EF, Siever LJ, Klar HM, et al: Serotonergic studies in patients with affective and personality disorders. Arch Gen Psychiatry 46:587–599, 1989

Coccaro EF, Astill JL, Herbert JL, et al: Fluoxetine treatment of impulsive aggression in DSM-III-R personality disorder patients (letter). J Clin Psychopharmacol 10:373–375, 1990

Convit A, Jaeger J, Lin SP, et al: Predicting assaultiveness in psychiatric inpatients: a pilot study. Hospital and Community Psychiatry 39:429–434, 1988

Cornelius JR, Soloff PH, Perel JM, et al: Fluoxetine trial in borderline personality disorder. Psychopharmacol Bull 26:151–154, 1990

Crowner ML, Stepcic F, Peric G, et al: Typology of patient-patient assaults detected by videocameras. Am J Psychiatry 151:1669–1672, 1994

Crowner ML, Peric G, Stepcic F, et al: Psychiatric patients' explanations for assaults. Psychiatr Serv 46:614–615, 1995

Czobor P, Volavka J, Meibach RC: Effect of risperidone on hostility in schizophrenia. J Clin Psychopharmacol 15:243–249, 1995

Dietch JT, Jennings RK: Aggressive dyscontrol in patients treated with benzodiazepines. J Clin Psychiatry 49:184–188, 1988

Drake RE, Ehrlich J: Suicide attempts associated with akathisia. Am J Psychiatry 142:499–501, 1985

Eichelman BS: Neurochemical and psychopharmacologic aspects of aggressive behavior. Annu Rev Med 41:149–158, 1990

Goldberg JF, Harrow M, Grossman LS: Recurrent affective syndromes in bipolar and unipolar mood disorders at follow-up. Br J Psychiatry 166:382–385, 1995

Grafman J, Schwab K, Warden D, et al: Frontal lobe injuries, violence, and aggression: a report of the Vietnam Head Injury Study. Neurology 46:1231–1238, 1996

Greendyke RM, Kanter DR, Schuster DB, et al: Propranolol treatment of assaultive patients with organic brain disease: a double-blind crossover, placebo-controlled study. J Nerv Ment Dis 174:290–294, 1986

Guy W: ECDEU Assessment Manual for Psychopharmacology—Revised (DHHS Publ No ADM 91-338). Rockville, MD, U.S. Department of Health, Education and Welfare, 1976

Hafner H, Boker W: Crimes of Violence by Mentally Abnormal Offenders: A Psychiatric and Epidemiological Study in the Federal German Republic. Cambridge, UK, Cambridge University Press, 1982

Herrera JN, Sramek JJ, Costa JF, et al: High potency neuroleptics and violence in schizophrenics. J Nerv Ment Dis 176:558–561, 1988

Keckich WA: Neuroleptics: violence as a manifestation of akathisia. JAMA 240:2185, 1978

Kemp R, David A: Psychological predictors of insight and compliance in psychotic patients. Br J Psychiatry 169:444–450, 1996

Kemp R, Hayward P, Applewhite G, et al: Compliance therapy in psychotic patients: randomised controlled trial. BMJ 312:345–349, 1996

Krakowski M, Volavka J, Brizer D: Psychopathology and violence: a review of the literature. Compr Psychiatry 27:131–148, 1986

Lau MA, Pihl RO: Provocation, acute alcohol intoxication, cognitive performance, and aggression. J Abnorm Psychol 104:150–155, 1995

Link BG, Stueve CA: Psychotic symptoms and the violent/illegal behavior of mental patients compared to community controls, in Violence and Mental Disorder: Developments in Risk Assessment. Edited by Monahan J, Steadman HJ. Chicago, IL, University of Chicago Press, 1994, pp 137–159

Lipinski JF, Zubenko G, Cohen BM, et al: Propranolol in the treatment of neuroleptic-induced akathisia. Am J Psychiatry 141:412–415, 1984

Malone RP, Rowan AB, Luebbert JF: Lithium for the treatment of aggression in conduct disorder. Poster presented at the 43rd annual meeting of the American Academy of Child and Adolescent Psychiatry, Philadelphia, PA, October 1996

Markovitz PJ, Calabrese JR, Schulz SC, et al: Fluoxetine in the treatment of borderline and schizotypal personality disorders. Am J Psychiatry 148:1064–1067, 1991

Martorano JT: Target symptoms in lithium carbonate therapy. Compr Psychiatry 13:533–537, 1972

Miller FA, Rampling D: Adverse effects of combined propranolol and chlorpromazine therapy. Am J Psychiatry 139:1198–1199, 1982

Myers KM, Dunner DL: Self and other directed violence on a closed acute-care ward. Psychiatr Q 56:178–188, 1984

Nemes ZC, Volavka J, Cooper TB, et al: Lithium and haloperidol (letter). Biol Psychiatry 21:568–569, 1986

Ratey JJ, Sorgi P, O'Driscoll GA, et al: Nadolol to treat aggression and psychiatric symptomatology in chronic psychiatric inpatients: a double-blind, placebo-controlled study. J Clin Psychiatry 53:41–46, 1992

Ratey JJ, Leveroni C, Kilmer D, et al: The effects of clozapine on severely aggressive psychiatric inpatients in a state hospital. J Clin Psychiatry 54:219–223, 1993

Schulte JL: Homicide and suicide associated with akathisia and haloperidol. American Journal of Forensic Psychiatry 6:3–7, 1985

Shear MK, Frances A, Weiden P: Suicide associated with akathisia and depot fluphenazine treatment. J Clin Psychopharmacol 3:235–236, 1983

Sheard MH: Effect of lithium in human aggression. Nature 230:113–114, 1971

Sheard MH: Lithium in the treatment of aggression. J Nerv Ment Dis 160:108–118, 1975

Sheard MH: Clinical pharmacology of aggressive behavior. Clin Neuropharmacol 7:173–183, 1984

Sheppard GP: High-dose propranolol in schizophrenia. Br J Psychiatry 134:470–476, 1979

Sobin P, Schneider L, McDernott H: Fluoxetine in the treatment of agitated dementia (letter). Am J Psychiatry 146:1636, 1989

Sorgi PJ, Ratey JJ, Polakoff S: Beta-blockers for the control of aggressive behaviors in patients with chronic schizophrenia. Am J Psychiatry 143:775–776, 1986

Tardiff K: Assessment and Management of Violent Patients, 2nd Edition. Washington, DC, American Psychiatric Press, 1996

Van Putten T, Sanders DG: Lithium in treatment failures. J Nerv Ment Dis 161:255–264, 1975

Van Putten T, Mutalipassi LR, Malkin MD: Phenothiazine-induced decompensation. Arch Gen Psychiatry 30:102–105, 1974

Vestral RE, Kornhauser DM, Hollifield JW: Inhibition of propranolol metabolism by chlorpromazine. Clin Pharmacol Ther 25:19–24, 1979

Volavka J: Neurobiology of Violence. Washington, DC, American Psychiatric Press, 1995

Volavka J, Mohammad Y, Vitrai J, et al: Characteristics of state hospital patients arrested for offenses committed during hospitalization. Psychiatr Serv 46:796–800, 1995a

Volavka J, Zito JM, Vitrai J, et al: Clozapine effects on hostility and aggression in schizophrenia (letter). J Clin Psychopharmacol 13:287–289, 1995b

Wilson W: Clinical review of clozapine treatment in a state hospital. Hospital and Community Psychiatry 43:700–703, 1992

CHAPTER 2

Assessment and Treatment of Abnormal Aggression in Children and Adolescents

Richard P. Malone, M.D.

Abnormal aggression in children and adolescents is a major public health problem (U.S. Department of Health and Human Services 1991) and one of the most common reasons for psychiatric referral. In some areas of the country, close to 25% of high school students report that they have been involved in physical fights (Centers for Disease Control and Prevention 1993). Abnormal aggression in childhood predicts abnormal aggression in adulthood (Loeber 1982, 1990; Loeber and Stouthamer-Loeber 1987; Robins 1966; Stewart and Kelso 1987) and can be a precursor of antisocial behavior in adulthood (Robins 1978).

A number of psychiatric disorders, including depressive disorders, psychotic disorders, and substance abuse, may be associated with increased aggression in those affected. In the case of these disorders, the treatment of the primary disorder often reduces the display of aggression. Aggression is also often present in children and adolescents who are diagnosed with conduct disorder. In DSM-IV (American Psychiatric Association 1994), aggressive behaviors constitute 9 of the 15 criteria for the diagnosis of conduct disorder. A subgroup of children and adolescents with conduct disorder demonstrate aggressive behavior that is serious and persistent (Loeber and Schmaling 1985a, 1985b; Stewart 1985).

Although a number of treatment approaches for reducing aggressive behavior, including psychopharmacological and behavioral approaches, have been studied (Campbell et al. 1982, 1984, 1995a; for review, see Kazdin 1987; Werry and Wollersheim 1989), few are well established. Overall, few controlled trials of psychotropic medication as a treatment for aggressive behavior in children and adolescents have been conducted. This is not surprising in that, except for the use of stimulant drugs in the treatment of attention-deficit disorders, there are few controlled clinical trials of psychoactive agents for most psychiatric disorders in children (Jensen et al. 1994). Consequently, an area of high national priority lies in increasing research on the safety and efficacy of psychotropic treatment in children (Institute of Medicine 1989). The paucity of pharmacological treatment research in this area is of concern, considering the high rate of drug treatment for aggressive behavior (Kaplan et al. 1994; Zito et al. 1994), particularly in light of the sociological issues and controversy surrounding the use of psychoactive agents in the young (Zito and Riddle 1995). Moreover, these medications are often administered clinically and for prolonged periods of time to children and adolescents who are aggressive.

The purpose of this chapter is twofold: to review the instruments that are available to assess aggression in children and adolescents and to review the results of controlled studies of pharmacological treatments for this problem in children and adolescents with conduct disorder.

Measures for the Assessment of Aggression

A number of measures have been developed to assess aggression, although the validity of many of these measures is not well established. Aggression is particularly difficult to measure because it is a relatively rare event, even in aggressive individuals. A number of instruments are discussed below, particularly as they relate to child and adolescent psychiatry. According to the way in which the information is obtained, measures can be subdivided as follows: observational measures, self-report measures, interview measures, and laboratory measures (Table 2–1).

Observational Measures

Several observational measures of aggression have been developed. The Overt Aggression Scale (OAS; Yudofsky et al. 1986) and the Aggression Questionnaire (Vitiello et al. 1990) are of particular interest for studies involving children and adolescents.

The OAS was originally developed as an instrument to measure aggression in hospitalized patients, including both child and adult populations. The OAS rates the behavioral frequency of four categories of aggression: 1) aggression against self, 2) aggression against others,

Table 2–1.　Measures of aggression

Measure	Type	Reference(s)
Buss-Durkee Hostility Inventory	Self-report	Buss and Durkee 1957
Spielberger Anger and Expression of Anger Inventory	Self-report	Spielberger 1988 (STAXI-HS); Spielberger et al. 1995 (STAXI-ETF)
Novaco Anger Inventory	Self-report	Novaco 1994
Anger, Irritability, and Aggression Questionnaire	Self-report	Coccaro et al. 1991
Buss-Perry Aggression Questionnaire	Self-report	Buss and Perry 1992
Child Behavior Checklist	Parent report	Achenbach 1991a
Youth Self-Report	Self-report	Achenbach 1991b
Retrospective Overt Aggression Scale	Interview (of observer)	Sorgi et al. 1991
Overt Aggression Scale Modified for Outpatients	Interview	Coccaro et al. 1991
Brown-Goodwin History of Lifetime Aggression	Interview	Brown et al. 1979
Life History of Aggression	Interview	Coccaro et al. 1996
Aggression Questionnaire	Observational	Vitiello et al. 1990
Overt Aggression Scale	Observational	Yudofsky et al. 1986
Staff Observation Aggression Scale	Observational	Palmstierna and Wistedt 1987
Modified Overt Aggression Scale	Observational	Kay et al. 1988
Social Dysfunction and Aggression Scale	Observational	Wistedt et al. 1990

Table 2–1. Measures of aggression (*continued*)

Measure	Type	Reference(s)
Scale for the Assessment of Aggression and Agitated Behaviors	Observational	Brizer et al. 1987
Children's Psychiatric Rating Scale	Observational	"Pharmacotherapy of Children" *Psychopharmacology Bulletin* 1973; "Rating Scales and Assessment Instruments" *Psychopharmacology Bulletin* 1985
Buss paradigm	Laboratory	Buss 1961
Taylor paradigm	Laboratory	Taylor 1967
Point Subtraction Aggression paradigm	Laboratory	Cherek 1981

3) aggression against objects, and 4) verbal aggression. Within each category, there are four levels of severity, each with a corresponding numeric score (see Silver and Yudofsky 1987). Reliability has been established, with intraclass correlation coefficients ranging from 0.5 to 0.97 for verbal aggression and 0.72 to 1.00 for physical aggression (Yudofsky et al. 1986). The OAS has been employed in a number of investigations (Cueva et al. 1996; Kafantaris et al. 1992; Malone et al. 1994b; Rifkin et al. 1989) as a measure of drug effect for the treatment of aggressive behavior in children and adolescents diagnosed with conduct disorder. The OAS has been modified by a number of authors for different uses, including for use with outpatients (OAS-Modified; Coccaro et al. 1991).

Classifying aggression into subtypes is essential for selecting patients who are most likely to respond to clinical drug treatment. In both animals and humans, aggression can be classified into the following two types: predatory and explosive/affective aggression (Eichelman 1990). The Aggression Questionnaire is a 16-item scale used to classify aggression into these types, as well as a mixed type. Eight of the items tap "predatory" aggression, and eight tap "affective" aggression. The Predatory-Affective Index, which is used to classify the aggression, is obtained by subtracting the score from the Affective items from the score from the Predatory items. It has been postulated that the "explosive" type of aggression is more responsive to drug treatment (Campbell et al. 1978, 1982, 1984, 1995a; Dostal 1972; Sheard et al. 1976). Although the Aggression Questionnaire is one of the few instruments used for typing aggression, few data exist regarding its usefulness. The Aggression Questionnaire has been modified for use in a self-report or interview format (Malone et al. 1996b). In this revision, each item is scored as follows: 0 = not true; 1 = partly true; and 2 = very true. In the case of children and adolescents, a parent or caregiver could be asked to complete the scale. Preliminary studies using this revision of the Aggression Questionnaire show that type of aggression may be related to treatment response (Malone et al. 1996b).

A number of other observational scales that measure aggression are used in child and adolescent psychiatry. The Children's Psychiatric Rating Scale is a 63-item scale developed by the Psychopharmacology Branch of the National Institute of Mental Health to rate childhood psychopathology ("Pharmacotherapy of Children" *Psychopharmacology Bulletin* 1973; "Rating Scales and Assessment Instruments" *Psychopharmacology Bulletin* 1985). Each of the items is rated from 1 (not present) to 7 (extremely severe). Although this scale contains factors covering a wide range of symptoms and behaviors, several items are particularly relevant in assessing treatment effect in children and adolescents with conduct disorder and aggression. Published studies (Campbell et al. 1982, 1984, 1995a) have shown that three factors of the Children's Psychiatric Rating Scale (composed of 10 items) indicate drug effect in treatment studies of aggression. The factors, along with the corresponding items, are 1) the hyperactivity factor (Item 3—fidgetiness, Item 4—hyperactivity, and Item 6—distractibility); 2) the aggression factor (Item 48—fighting with peers, Item 49—bullying, and Item 50—temper outbursts); and 3) the hostility factor (Item 10—negative, uncooperative, Item 11—angry affect, Item 20—lability of affect, and Item 25—loud voice).

Several of the Conners rating scales may be of use in measuring aggression. The IOWA Conners (Loney and Milich 1982) is a 10-item scale that was developed from earlier parent and teacher versions of the Conners rating scales (see Guy 1976). This scale, which has separate hyperactivity and aggression factors, has been used in studies of hyperactive and aggressive children as a measure of drug effect (Gadow et al. 1990).

Self-Report Measures

The Buss-Durkee Hostility Inventory (BDHI; Buss and Durkee 1957), one of the earliest developed self-report measures of aggression, remains one of the most used measures. Scores from the BDHI have been shown to correlate with biological measures (Castrogiovanni et al. 1994; Coccaro et al. 1989, 1996; Siever et al. 1992). The BDHI is limited in that the answers are true/false only. The Buss-Perry Aggression Questionnaire (Buss and Perry 1992) is an improvement of the BDHI in that it employs a Likert scale for a broader range of responses. Another modification of the BDHI, called the Anger, Irritability, and Aggression Questionnaire (Coccaro et al. 1991), employs both Likert scoring and a time frame (which is helpful in treatment trials).

The Youth Self-Report (Achenbach 1991b) is a 112-item self-report questionnaire designed for children ages 11–18 years. Scoring is standardized for age and sex and includes a Total Problem score, an Internalizing Problem score, an Externalizing Problem score, and a number of derived Narrow-Band Syndromes. In a controlled trial of lithium as a treatment for aggression, placebo baseline responders differed from nonresponders on the Youth Self-Report Externalizing Problem score (Malone et al. 1994a). A related measure, the Child Behavior Checklist—Parent Version, has been shown to correlate with biological measures (Birmaher et al. 1990; Stoff et al. 1987).

Interview Measures

The Brown-Goodwin History of Lifetime Aggression (Brown et al. 1979) was devised for military populations to give a life history of aggression. Scores from the nine items range from 0 (no events) to 4 (multiple events). Scores from this measure correlate with biological measures (low levels of 5-hydroxyindoleacetic acid) associated with aggression in both adults (Brown et al. 1982) and children (Castellanos et al. 1994; Kruesi et al. 1990). A revision of this measure (Coccaro et al. 1992) was also shown to be correlated with biological measures (Coccaro et al. 1996).

Laboratory Measures

Two laboratory measures, the Buss (1961) and the Taylor (1967) paradigms, have been widely employed in human aggression research (Bernstein et al. 1987). In the Buss paradigm, the subject is instructed to reward or punish a confederate for task performance. The punishment is an electric shock controlled by the subject, who can vary its intensity and duration. In the Taylor paradigm, the subject engages in a reaction-time competition with a confederate. Ostensibly, the loser of the competition is shocked with the level of shock set by the winner. In these paradigms, the measure of aggression is the level of shock the subject chooses to deliver to the confederate (see Bernstein et al. 1987 for a discussion of validity of these measures). Scores from these paradigms correlate with aggression in children (for review, see Cherek et al. 1996).

Another laboratory measure, the Point Subtraction Aggression paradigm (Cherek 1981), was found to be sensitive to the effects of stimulants in children (Casat et al. 1995). This paradigm reportedly measures two kinds of aggression: instrumental (goal-directed) aggression and hostile (reactive) aggression. In a controlled study involving six children (ages 8–11 years) with a DSM-III-R diagnosis of attention-deficit hyperactivity disorder, administration of one dose of methylphenidate (0.6 mg/kg) was associated with a decrease in aggressive responding.

Additionally, a laboratory task based on a pinball game was devised to measure instrumental and hostile aggression (Atkins and Stoff 1993; Atkins et al. 1993). On this task, aggressive children, both with and without attention-deficit disorder, had higher rates of instrumental aggression than nonaggressive healthy control subjects, whereas only the aggressive children with attention-deficit disorder had higher rates of hostile aggression than the control subjects. These results suggest that a laboratory measure such as the pinball task may be useful in typing aggression in children.

Pharmacotherapy of Aggression

Medications

A number of medications have been studied for their efficacy in reducing aggression in children and adolescents (Table 2–2). The purpose of this section is to review the controlled trials of medications in children and adolescents who have a primary problem with aggression related to a disruptive disorder but who do not have a psychotic disorder, affective disorder, or mental retardation. Over the years, a number of different classification systems have been used in making psychiatric diagnoses in children and adolescents, making it difficult to determine which DSM-IV diagnoses would apply to the subjects described in the various studies. In the most recent studies, in which DSM-IV criteria were used, the subjects were diagnosed with conduct disorder or, at times, attention-deficit hyperactivity disorder.

Anticonvulsants

Phenytoin (diphenylhydantoin), which is classified as an anticonvulsant drug, was one of the earliest drugs investigated in controlled trials for efficacy in treating aggression. These controlled trials followed open reports of efficacy for this medication in treating aggression. The subjects of these studies were said to be delinquent youths with mixed behavioral disorders. Despite the fact that there were uncontrolled reports of efficacy, none of the controlled trials found diphenylhydantoin to be efficacious (Table 2–2). The dosages employed in these studies were 200 mg/day of diphenylhydantoin, though in one study dosage was adjusted to attain serum diphenylhydantoin levels above 10 µg/mL. Untoward effects of medication treatment included possible worsening of behavior and mood (Lefkowitz 1969).

Another anticonvulsant, carbamazepine, has also been investigated as a treatment for aggression in children and adolescents. Groh (1976) and Puente (1976) conducted controlled trials of carbamazepine for the treatment of disruptive behavior; however, the significance of their findings is difficult to interpret. It is not clear that aggression in particular was measured in these studies or that carbamazepine was associated with a reduction of aggression, although it seems that there was improvement in other areas such as irritable affect. On the basis of the promise of potential benefit for treating aggression indicated by these earlier

Table 2–2. Drugs in the treatment of aggression: controlled trials

Drug(s) (dosage)	N	Ages (years)	Sex[a]	Diagnosis	Design[b]	Setting	Results	Reference
Anticonvulsants								
Diphenylhydantoin[c] (200 mg)	50	13–16 (mean = 14.11)	M	Delinquent behavior	DB, PC (76 days)	Residential	Not effective; placebo = diphenyl-hydantoin	Lefkowitz 1969
Diphenylhydantoin[c] (serum level > 10 µg/mL)	17	5–14 (mean = 9)	14 M, 3 F	Mixed behavioral disorders	DB, PC crossover (9 weeks)	Outpatient	Not effective	Looker and Conners 1970
Diphenylhydantoin[c] (200 mg/day), methylphenidate (20 mg/day)	43	9–14 (mean = 12)	M	Delinquent behavior	DB, PC (2 weeks)	Residential	Not effective	Conners et al. 1971
Carbamazepine (dosage not stated)	20	8–14	Not stated	Nonepileptic, normal intelligence	DB, PC crossover	Not stated	Unclear	Groh 1976
Carbamazepine (200–300 mg/day)	27	5–13 (mean = 8.7)	12 M, 15 F	Mixed behavioral disorders[d]	DB, PC crossover	Unclear	Unclear	Puente 1976
Carbamazepine (400–800 mg/day)	22	5.3–11.7	20 M, 2 F	Conduct disorder	DB, PC	Inpatient	Not effective	Cueva et al. 1996

Table 2–2. Drugs in the treatment of aggression: controlled trials (continued)

Drug(s) (dosage)	N	Ages (years)	Sex[a]	Diagnosis	Design[b]	Setting	Results	Reference
Stimulants								
Dextroamphetamine, levoamphetamine (mean = 28.5–34.5 mg/day)	11	Not stated	Not stated	Mixed	DB, PC crossover	Not stated	Effective	Arnold et al. 1973
Methylphenidate (up to 60 mg/day), dextroamphetamine (up to 40 mg/day)	18	5–10 (mean = 8.5)	15 M, 3 F	Hyperactivity, aggression	DB, PC crossover (about 9 days per drug)	Inpatient	Effective	Winsberg et al. 1974
Dextroamphetamine (15–30 mg/day)	10	Mean (SD) = 9.6 (1.6)	M	ADDH	DB, PC crossover	Inpatient	Effective	Amery et al. 1984
Methylphenidate (0.3 or 0.6 mg/kg per day)	11	5.9–11.9	M	ADDH and aggression	DB, PC crossover	Outpatient	Effective	Gadow et al. 1990
Methylphenidate (20–60 mg/day)	9	13–16 (mean = 14.4)	M	CD, ADDH	DB, PC crossover (3 open)	Inpatient and outpatient	Not effective	Kaplan et al. 1990

Table 2-2. Drugs in the treatment of aggression: controlled trials (*continued*)

Drug(s) (dosage)	N	Ages (years)	Sex[a]	Diagnosis	Design[b]	Setting	Results	Reference
Antipsychotics								
Perphenazine (≤16 mg/day)	56	10–15	M	Delinquent behavior	DB, PC parallel (partial)	Residential	Drug = placebo	Molling et al. 1962
Haloperidol (0.05 mg/kg per day)	16	4–15	10 M, 6 F	Mixed behavioral disorders	DB, PC crossover (6 weeks)	Inpatient and outpatient	Effective	Barker and Fraser 1968
Haloperidol (1–3 mg/day)	12	7–12	Not given	Mixed behavioral disorders	DB, PC crossover	Inpatient	Effective	Cunningham et al. 1968
Haloperidol (1–6 mg/day), lithium (500–2,000 mg/day)	61	5.2–12.9	57 M, 4 F	CD, unsocialized aggressive	DB, PC parallel	Inpatient	Both effective	Campbell et al. 1984
Molindone (26.8 mg/day), thioridazine (mean = 169.9 mg/day)	31	6–11	M	CD, unsocialized aggressive	DB, PC parallel (8 weeks)	Inpatient	Both effective	Greenhill et al. 1985

Table 2–2.   Drugs in the treatment of aggression: controlled trials (continued)

Drug(s) (dosage)	N	Ages (years)	Sex[a]	Diagnosis	Design[b]	Setting	Results	Reference
Lithium								
Lithium (1,212–1,691 mg/day)	66	16–24	M	Aggression	DB, PC	Prison	Effective	Sheard et al. 1976
Lithium (500–2,000 mg/day), haloperidol (1–6 mg/day)	61	5.2–12.9	57 M, 4 F	CD, unsocial-ized aggressive	DB, PC parallel	Inpatient	Both effective	Campbell et al. 1984
Lithium (600–1,800 mg/day)	50	5.1–12.0	46 M, 4 F	CD, unsocial-ized aggressive	DB, PC parallel	Inpatient	Effective	Campbell et al. 1995a
Lithium (dosage adjusted for serum level = 0.6–1.2 mEq/L)	33	12–17	14 M, 19 F	CD	DB, PC parallel (3 weeks)	Inpatient	Not effective	Rifkin et al. 1989
Lithium (dosage adjusted for serum level = 0.6–1.2 mEq/L), methylpheni-date (up to 60 mg/day)	35	6–15	Not stat-ed	ADHD	DB, PC parallel	Outpatient	Lithium not effective	Klein 1991

Note. ADDH = attention deficit disorder with hyperactivity; ADHD = attention-deficit hyperactivity disorder; CD = conduct disorder.

[a]M = males; F = females. [b]DB = double-blind; PC = placebo-controlled. [c]Now called phenytoin.
[d]Included 11 individuals with "mental deficiency" or brain damage.

reports, a more recent double-blind, placebo-controlled study was conducted (Cueva et al. 1996). The subjects were 22 children (both males and females), ages 5–11 years, who were diagnosed with conduct disorder, solitary aggressive type (DSM-III-R [American Psychiatric Association 1987]). All had long histories of explosive aggression. Optimal carbamazepine dosages ranged from 400 to 800 mg/day (mean dosage = 683 mg/day), and serum carbamazepine levels ranged from 4.98 to 9.1 µg/mL (mean = 6.81 µg/mL). In this study, carbamazepine was not found to be superior to placebo. Untoward effects that were found more commonly with drug than with placebo included transient leukopenia, rash, dizziness, drowsiness, headache, blurred vision, and nausea (Cueva et al. 1996).

Thus, controlled studies of anticonvulsants as a treatment to reduce aggression in children and adolescents have not clearly demonstrated efficacy for this usage. Further research in this area is indicated.

Stimulants

The effectiveness of stimulants in the treatment of aggression has also been explored. The subjects for these studies are described as hyperactive and aggressive, although it is not clear that they would meet the DSM-IV criteria for conduct disorder. Unfortunately, the sample sizes in the studies are small; this makes it difficult to assess the significance of the results. Overall, the reported dosages for methylphenidate ranged up to 60 mg/day and those for dextroamphetamine ranged up to 40 mg/day. Although untoward effects were not reported in many of these studies, when they were reported, stimulant usage was associated with anorexia, insomnia (Winsberg et al. 1974), weight loss, confusion, nervousness, and abdominal cramps (Eisenberg et al. 1963; Korey 1944). Despite the limitations of these studies, stimulants show promise as a treatment for aggression, particularly when the subjects have a primary diagnosis of attention-deficit/hyperactivity disorder (ADHD). It is not clear, however, that stimulants are effective for treating severe aggression in children and adolescents with a primary diagnosis of conduct disorder.

Antipsychotics

Almost since the time they were introduced, antipsychotics have been used in children and adolescents with conduct disorder to reduce aggression. Haloperidol, a high-potency antipsychotic, is the one that has been most studied as a treatment for aggression. Haloperidol dosages reported in these studies (Table 2–2) ranged from 1 to 6 mg/day. Barker and Fraser (1968) and

Cunningham et al. (1968) reported on small samples of children and adolescents with mixed behavioral disorders in studies that used crossover designs. In Barker and Fraser's study, among the inclusion criteria was the presence of hyperactivity and aggression. Their sample included children with histories of seizure disorders and autism. It is not clear how their results pertain to children with conduct disorder. The largest study involving haloperidol for the treatment of aggression was that of Campbell et al. (1984), in which the use of lithium was also examined (see later in this section). In this study, both haloperidol and lithium were found to be effective, although fewer side effects were experienced by subjects treated with lithium than by those treated with haloperidol (see also Platt et al. 1984). Overall, untoward effects with haloperidol included sedation, dystonic reactions, tremor, and drooling.

In a study comparing the low-potency antipsychotic thioridazine, with molindone, Greenhill et al. (1985) found both to be effective for reducing aggression (Table 2–2). However, side effects for the two drugs were different. The molindone-treated subjects exhibited more dystonic reactions and needed more dosage changes because of toxicity. The thioridazine-treated subjects had higher rates of sedation, gastric upset, headache, poor compliance, and weight gain.

Although most studies of antipsychotics in the treatment of aggression have been positive, there have been negative reports. The study by Molling et al. (1962) is particularly interesting because it emphasizes important methodological problems encountered in aggression research—namely, that the rate of aggression fluctuates over time and there can be an apparently significant positive treatment effect, even with placebo. During the first month of the study, baseline ratings were obtained for the children in a medication-free condition. Following this baseline period, the children were divided into three experimental groups: the first group received perphenazine, the second group received placebo, and the third group did not receive any study medication or placebo. During the baseline drug-free period, the ratings for all three groups initially improved and then gradually reverted. During the experimental treatment period, both the perphenazine and placebo groups showed significant improvement in aggressive behavior from baseline, whereas the group that did not receive drug or placebo had worsening of behavior. Thus, the effect of placebo on significantly disruptive behavior should not be overlooked.

Lithium

Since its introduction in 1949 (Cade 1949), lithium has been shown to be effective in the treatment of mania, a syndrome in which patients often display verbal and physical aggression. Sheard conducted a series of placebo-controlled investigations of lithium in the treatment of chronically impulsive and aggressive young adult prisoners, employing both single-blind (Sheard 1971, 1975) and double-blind designs (Sheard et al. 1976). In his double-blind and placebo-controlled study, the subjects were 66 male prisoners, ranging in age from 16 to 24 years (mean age $\pm$ SD = 19.4 $\pm$ 1.76 for subjects taking lithium and 19.5 $\pm$ 1.49 for subjects taking placebo). Lithium was administered for 1–3 months at average weekly dosages ranging from 1,212 to 1,691 mg/day. Corresponding 24-hour serum lithium levels ranged from 0.68 to 0.80 mEq/L. These levels were 24-hour levels because the study employed once-daily lithium dosing. With twice-daily dosing, levels would have been 12-hour levels. Most likely, they would have been higher than 24-hour levels. The results of this study were highly suggestive of efficacy, despite methodological flaws, including the variable length of treatment periods for subjects and the reliance on routine institutional records as the main measure of aggression.

In all, four double-blind, placebo-controlled studies of lithium as a treatment for aggressive behavior in conduct disorder have been conducted (for review, see Campbell et al. 1995b). Their results are not in agreement. Campbell et al. (1984, 1995a) reported on two major lithium studies that were double-blind, placebo-controlled and used random assignment. Both were conducted in an inpatient setting. In the first study (Campbell et al. 1984), lithium was compared with haloperidol in 61 aggressive subjects with conduct disorder ages 5–12 years (mean age = 9 years). Following a 2-week baseline period, subjects were randomized to either lithium (500 to 2,000 mg/day; optimal serum levels of 0.32–1.51 mEq/L; mean serum level = 0.99 mEq/L), haloperidol (1–6 mg/day; mean = 2.95 mg/day), or placebo for 4 weeks. Overall, the two drugs (lithium and haloperidol) were significantly superior to placebo in reducing behavioral symptoms. Except for side effects, the drugs were not significantly different from each other. Haloperidol produced significantly more side effects than lithium. In the second study (Campbell et al. 1995a), lithium and placebo were compared in 50 aggressive subjects with conduct disorder ages 5–12 years (mean age = 9.4 years). They were treated with the study drug for a period of 6 weeks. Optimal daily dosages of lithium ranged from 600 to 1,800 mg (median = 1,248 mg; mean serum level = 1.12 mEq/L). Lithium was again found to be effective in reducing aggressive behavior in this second study. Lithium side effects were examined in the subjects from both of these studies combined (Silva et al. 1992). Enuresis, fatigue, ataxia, decreased motor activity, diplopia, and dysarthria were among the side effects found exclusively in subjects receiving lithium. A number of other side effects were found in both lithium and placebo subjects. Among these, nausea, vomiting, and tremor were significantly more common in subjects taking lithium than in placebo subjects. Others, including headache, stomachache, sedation, diarrhea, and polyuria, were not significantly different in lithium- and placebo-treated subjects. Side effects were more common in younger children (Campbell et al. 1991).

The findings of Campbell et al. (1984, 1995a) were not replicated in the other two double-blind, placebo-controlled studies. Rifkin et al. (1989) conducted a double-blind, placebo-controlled trial of lithium in 33 hospitalized patients (ages 12–17 years) diagnosed with conduct disorder who exhibited a behavioral profile of aggressiveness. However, the 2-week treatment trial in this study was insufficient. Consequently, the study is not helpful in evaluating the efficacy of lithium as a treatment for aggression. In an interim account, Klein (1991) reported on 35 outpatients with DSM-III-R conduct disorder (ages 6–15 years) who were randomized to lithium (serum levels ranging from 0.6 to 1.2 mEq/L), methylphenidate (up to 60 mg/day), or placebo for a period of 5 weeks. Lithium was found to be ineffective as a treatment for aggressive behavior, whereas methylphenidate was found to be effective. Unlike the subjects in the studies by Campbell et al., the subjects in the study by Klein did not have histories of severe and explosive aggression. Also, Campbell et al. conducted studies in an inpatient setting, whereas Klein conducted the study in an outpatient setting. The difference in diagnosis and setting may select for very different populations and levels of pathology. Regardless, the efficacy of lithium for reducing aggression in adolescents still needs to be established, not only in the inpatient setting but in the outpatient setting as well.

The question of efficacy in an older population is being addressed in an ongoing 6-week double-blind, placebo-controlled trial (Malone et al. 1996c). Following a 2-week single-blind placebo baseline period, subjects with conduct disorder (DSM-III-R) are randomized to a 4-week double-blind treatment period in which they are administered either lithium or placebo. Preliminary results from this study are important in that they suggest that lithium is efficacious in reducing aggression in an older sample that includes adolescents. In a previous report (McGuffin et al. 1994) from this study, it was noted that at optimal dosage no detrimental cognitive effects on the Mazes Test of the Wechsler Intelligence Scale for Children—Revised and on the Trail Making Test (Forms A and B) occurred with lithium treatment. It was also noted that the subjects taking lithium improved more on their Mazes Test scores than did the placebo-treated subjects, suggesting that the lithium-treated subjects developed a less impulsive approach to the task. A dose prediction method (Cooper and Simpson 1976; Cooper et al. 1973) was used safely to attain therapeutic serum levels of lithium (Malone et al. 1995). Other preliminary analyses suggested that placebo baseline responders had less severe disturbance and less hyperactivity (Malone et al. 1996a).

Long-Term Treatment

While our knowledge regarding the short-term use of the aforementioned medications in children is limited, even less is known about the long-term safety and efficacy of these treatments. There is only one double-blind, placebo-controlled study of lithium as a long-term treatment for aggressive behavior in conduct disorder, but because of its small sample size, the results were inconclusive (Campbell et al. 1995b; Silva et al. 1991). In that study, children who responded to lithium during a short-term controlled trial were randomized to outpatient treatment with lithium or placebo under double-blind conditions for a period of 6 months. Aggressive symptoms decreased in both the lithium and placebo groups. It is important that lithium was found to be a safe treatment during the 6-month study period. Delong and Aldershof (1987) reported on their experience with 196 children with a variety of diagnoses who were treated with lithium for periods ranging from 1 to 10 years. They reported that only one of the children who received treatment had a complication that required lithium discontinuation; this child had hypothyroidism, which resolved when lithium was discontinued. These limited reports on long-term lithium treatment in children suggest that lithium can be administered safely, although more study on its safety is needed.

There are no studies on the long-term use of any of the antipsychotics as a treatment for aggression in children and adolescents. However, the effects of long-term treatment with haloperidol in children with autism have been reported (Campbell et al. 1988; Perry et al. 1989). In this study, haloperidol remained safe and efficacious with long-term use, although there was a definite risk of developing dyskinesias. It is not known whether the risk of developing dyskinesias is the same when haloperidol is used to reduce aggression in children and adolescents with conduct disorder. Given that aggressive conduct disorder is a chronic condition and may require long-term treatment, lithium is a preferable treatment. The antipsychotics have more adverse cognitive side effects than lithium (Platt et al. 1984), and they carry the risk of dyskinesias (Campbell et al. 1988).

The long-term usage of stimulants and carbamazepine to treat aggression has not been studied. In the long-term use of these agents for attention-deficit/hyperactivity disorder, the effects on weight and height are of concern (Safer and Allen 1973; Safer et al. 1972; for review, see Klein and Bessler 1992), although the effect on height is controversial (Klein and Mannuzza 1988; Vincent et al. 1990). Likewise, long-term administration of carbamazepine to children and adolescents for seizures has generally been safe (Dreyer 1976).

Conclusion

Although aggression in children and adolescents is a serious public health problem and is often the reason for referral for psychiatric services, there are few well-established treatments for this behavior. Several instruments have been used in this research to date, including the Overt Aggression Scale and the Children's Psychiatric Rating Scale. Many children and adolescents who display aggression are treated with pharmacotherapy, although there are few well-designed studies to support this practice. The neuroleptics and lithium are the better-studied drugs for the treatment of aggression in children and adolescents, though even for these treatments there are limited data to guide the clinician. Clearly, when neuroleptics are used, the clinician must weigh the risk to the child or adolescent of developing dyskinesias. Although there is support for the use of lithium in hospitalized children to treat aggression, there is a paucity of data regarding its use in outpatients. More research is needed to guide the clinician in the treatment of this difficult and common problem.

References

Achenbach TM: Manual for the Child Behavior Checklist/4–18 and 1991 Profile. Burlington, VT, University of Vermont, Department of Psychiatry, 1991a

Achenbach TM: Manual for the Youth Self-Report and 1991 Profile. Burlington, VT, University of Vermont, Department of Psychiatry, 1991b

American Psychiatric Association: Diagnostic and Statistical Manual of Mental Disorders, 3rd Edition, Revised. Washington, DC, American Psychiatric Association, 1987

American Psychiatric Association: Diagnostic and Statistical Manual of Mental Disorders, 4th Edition. Washington, DC, American Psychiatric Association, 1994

Amery B, Minichiello MD, Brown GL: Aggression in hyperactive boys: response to d-amphetamine. J Am Acad Child Adolesc Psychiatry 23:291–294, 1984

Arnold LE, Kirilcuk V, Corson SA, et al: Levoamphetamine and dextro-amphetamine: differential effect on aggression and hyperkinesis in children and dogs. Am J Psychiatry 130:165–170, 1973

Atkins MS, Stoff DM: Instrumental and hostile aggression in childhood disruptive behavior disorders. J Abnorm Child Psychol 21:165–178, 1993

Atkins MS, Stoff DM, Osborne ML, et al: Distinguishing instrumental and hostile aggression: does it make a difference? J Abnorm Child Psychol 21:355–365, 1993

Barker P, Fraser IA: A controlled trial of haloperidol in children. Br J Psychiatry 114:855–857, 1968

Bernstein S, Richardson D, Hammock G: Convergent and discriminant validity of the Taylor and Buss measures of physical aggression. Aggressive Behavior 13:15–24, 1987

Birmaher B, Stanley M, Greenhill L, et al: Platelet imipramine binding in children and adolescents with impulsive behavior. J Am Acad Child Adolesc Psychiatry 29:914–918, 1990

Brizer DA, Convit A, Krakowski M, et al: A rating scale for reporting violence on psychiatric wards. Hospital and Community Psychiatry 38:769–770, 1987

Brown GL, Goodwin FK, Ballenger JC, et al: Aggression in humans correlates with cerebrospinal fluid amine metabolites. Psychiatry Res 1:131–139, 1979

Brown GL, Ebert MH, Goyer PF, et al: Aggression, suicide, and serotonin: relationships to CSF amine metabolites. Am J Psychiatry 139:741–746, 1982

Buss AH: The Psychology of Aggression. New York, Wiley, 1961

Buss AH, Durkee A: An inventory for assessing different types of hostility. Journal of Consulting Psychology 21:343–349, 1957

Buss AH, Perry M: The Aggression Questionnaire. Journal of Personality and Psychology 63:452–459, 1992

Cade JFJ: Lithium salts in the treatment of psychotic excitement. Med J Aust 36:349–352, 1949

Campbell M, Schulman D, Rapoport JL: The current status of lithium therapy in child and adolescent psychiatry. Journal of the American Academy of Child Psychiatry 17:717–720, 1978

Campbell M, Cohen IL, Small AM: Drugs in aggressive behavior. Journal of the American Academy of Child Psychiatry 21:107–117, 1982

Campbell M, Small AM, Green WH, et al: Behavioral efficacy of haloperidol and lithium carbonate: a comparison in hospitalized aggressive children with conduct disorder. Arch Gen Psychiatry 41:650–656, 1984

Campbell M, Adams P, Perry R, et al: Tardive and withdrawal dyskinesia in autistic children: a prospective study. Psychopharmacol Bull 24:251–255, 1988

Campbell M, Silva RR, Kafantaris V, et al: Predictors of side effects associated with lithium administration in children. Psychopharmacol Bull 27:373–380, 1991

Campbell M, Adams PB, Small AM, et al: Lithium in hospitalized aggressive children with conduct disorder: a double-blind and placebo-controlled study. J Am Acad Child Adolesc Psychiatry 34:445–453, 1995a

Campbell M, Kafantaris V, Cueva JE: An update on the use of lithium carbonate in aggressive children and adolescents with conduct disorder. Psychopharmacol Bull 31:93–102, 1995b

Casat CD, Pearson DA, Van Davelaar MJ, et al: Methylphenidate effects on a laboratory aggression measure in children with ADHD. Psychopharmacol Bull 31:353–356, 1995

Castellanos FX, Elia J, Kruesi MJ, et al: Cerebrospinal fluid monoamine metabolites in boys with attention-deficit hyperactivity disorder. Psychiatry Res 52:305–316, 1994

Castrogiovanni P, Capone MR, Maremmani I, et al: Platelet serotonergic markers and aggressive behaviour in healthy subjects. Neuropsychobiology 29:105–107, 1994

Centers for Disease Control and Prevention: Violence-related attitudes and behaviors of high school students—New York City, 1992. MMWR Morb Mortal Wkly Rep 42(40):773–777, 1993

Cherek DR: Effects of smoking different doses of nicotine on human aggressive behavior. Psychopharmacology (Berl) 75:339–349, 1981

Cherek DR, Schnapp W, Moeller FG, et al: Aggressive responding of violent and non-violent male parolees under laboratory conditions. Aggressive Behavior 22:27–36, 1996

Coccaro EF, Siever LJ, Klar HM, et al: Serotonergic studies in patients with affective and personality disorders. Arch Gen Psychiatry 46: 587–599, 1989

Coccaro EF, Harvey PD, Kupsaw-Lawrence E, et al: Development of neuropharmacologically based behavioral assessments of impulsive aggressive behavior. J Neuropsychiatry Clin Neurosci 3(suppl 2): S44-S51, 1991

Coccaro EF, Kavoussi RJ, Lesser J: Self- and other-directed human aggression: the role of the central serotonergic system. Int Clin Psychopharmacol 6(56):70–83, 1992

Coccaro EF, Kavoussi RJ, Sheline YI, et al: Impulsive aggression in personality disorder correlates with tritiated paroxetine binding in the platelet. Arch Gen Psychiatry 53:531–536, 1996

Conners CK, Kramer R, Rothschild GH, et al: Treatment of young delinquent boys with diphenylhydantoin sodium and methylphenidate. Arch Gen Psychiatry 24:156–160, 1971

Cooper TB, Simpson GM: The 24-hour serum lithium level as a prognosticator of dosage requirements: a 2-year follow-up study. Am J Psychiatry 133:440–443, 1976

Cooper TB, Bergner PE, Simpson GM: The 24-hour serum lithium level as a prognosticator of dosage requirements. Am J Psychiatry 130: 601–603, 1973

Cueva JE, Overall JE, Small AM, et al: Carbamazepine in aggressive children with conduct disorder: a double-blind and placebo-controlled study. J Am Acad Child Adolesc Psychiatry 35:480–490, 1996

Cunningham MA, Pillai V, Blachford Rogers WJ: Haloperidol in the treatment of children with severe behaviour disorders. Br J Psychiatry 114:845–854, 1968

Delong GR, Aldershof AL: Long-term experience with lithium treatment in childhood: correlation with clinical diagnosis. J Am Acad Child Adolesc Psychiatry 26:389–394, 1987

Dostal T: Antiaggressive effects of lithium salts in mentally retarded adolescents, in Depressive States in Childhood and Adolescence. Edited by Annell AL. Stockholm, Almqvist & Wiksell, 1972, pp 491–498

Dreyer R: The long-term administration of anti-epileptic agents, with particular reference to pharmacotoxicological aspects, in Epileptic Seizures–Behaviour–Pain. Edited by Birkmayer W. Bern, Switzerland, Hans Huber, 1976, pp 76–97

Eichelman BS: Neurochemical and psychopharmacologic aspects of aggressive behavior. Annu Rev Med 41:149–158, 1990

Eisenberg L, Lachman R, Molling PA, et al: A psychopharmacologic experiment in a training school for delinquent boys: methods, problems, findings. Am J Orthopsychiatry 33:431–447, 1963

Gadow KD, Nolan EE, Sverd J, et al: Methylphenidate in aggressive-hyperactive boys, I: effects on peer aggression in public school settings. J Am Acad Child Adolesc Psychiatry 29:710–718, 1990

Greenhill LL, Solomon M, Pleak R, et al: Molindone hydrochloride treatment of hospitalized children with conduct disorder. J Clin Psychiatry 46 (no 8, sec 2):20–25, 1985

Groh C: The psychotropic effect of Tegretol in non-epileptic children, with particular reference to the drug's indications, in Epileptic Seizures–Behaviour–Pain. Edited by Birkmayer W. Bern, Switzerland, Hans Huber, 1976, pp 259–263

Guy W: ECDEU Assessment Manual for Psychopharmacology—Revised (DHEW Publ No ADM-76–338). Rockville, MD, U.S. Department of Health, Education and Welfare, 1976

Institute of Medicine: Research on Children and Adolescents With Mental, Behavioral and Developmental Disorders: Mobilizing a National Initiative. Washington, DC, National Academy Press, 1989, pp 1–11

Jensen PS, Vitiello B, Leonard H, et al: Design and methodology issues for clinical treatment trials in children and adolescents. Psychopharmacol Bull 30:3–8, 1994

Kafantaris V, Campbell M, Padron-Gayol MV, et al: Carbamazepine in hospitalized aggressive conduct disordered children: an open pilot study. Psychopharmacol Bull 28:193–199, 1992

Kaplan SL, Busner J, Kupietz S, et al: Effects of methylphenidate on adolescents with aggressive conduct disorder and ADDH: a preliminary report. J Am Acad Child Adolesc Psychiatry 29:719–723, 1990

Kaplan SL, Simms RM, Busner J: Prescribing practices of outpatient child psychiatrists. J Am Acad Child Adolesc Psychiatry 33:35–44, 1994

Kay SR, Wolkenfeld F, Murrill LM: Profiles of aggression among psychiatric patients, I: nature and prevalence. J Nerv Ment Dis 176:539–546, 1988

Kazdin AE: Conduct Disorders in Childhood and Adolescence, Vol 9: Developmental Clinical Psychology and Psychiatry Series. Newbury Park, CA, Sage, 1987

Klein RG: Preliminary results: lithium effects in conduct disorders, in CME Syllabus and Proceedings Summary, Symposium 2, American Psychiatric Association, 144th Annual Meeting, New Orleans, LA, May 11–16, 1991. Washington, DC, American Psychiatric Association, 1991, pp 119–120

Klein RG, Bessler AW: Stimulant side effects in children, in Adverse Effects of Psychotropic Drugs. Edited by Kane JM, Lieberman JA. New York, Guilford, 1992, pp 470–496

Klein RG, Mannuzza S: Hyperactive boys almost grown up. Arch Gen Psychiatry 45:1131–1134, 1988

Korey SR: The effects of benzedrine sulfate on the behavior of psychopathic and neurotic juvenile delinquents. Psychiatr Q 18:127–137, 1944

Kruesi MJP, Rapoport JL, Hamburger S, et al: Cerebrospinal fluid monoamine metabolites, aggression, and impulsivity in disruptive behavior disorders of children and adolescents. Arch Gen Psychiatry 47:419–426, 1990

Lefkowitz MM: Effects of diphenylhydantoin on disruptive behavior: study of male delinquents. Arch Gen Psychiatry 20:643–651, 1969

Loeber R: The stability of antisocial and delinquent child behavior: a review. Child Dev 53:1431-1446, 1982

Loeber R: Development and risk factors of juvenile antisocial behavior and delinquency. Clin Psychol Rev 10:1–41, 1990

Loeber R, Schmaling KB: Empirical evidence for overt and covert patterns of antisocial conduct problems: a meta-analysis. J Abnorm Child Psychol 13:337–352, 1985a

Loeber R, Schmaling KB: The utility of differentiating between mixed and pure forms of antisocial child behavior. J Abnorm Child Psychol 13:315–336, 1985b

Loeber R, Stouthamer-Loeber M: Prediction, in Handbook of Juvenile Delinquency. Edited by Quay HC. New York, Wiley, 1987, pp 325–382

Loney J, Milich RS: Hyperactivity, inattention, and aggression in clinical practice, in Advances in Developmental and Behavioral Pediatrics, Vol 3. Edited by Wolraich M, Routh DK. Greenwich, CT, JAI Press, 1982, pp 113–147

Looker A, Conners CK: Diphenylhydantoin in children with severe temper tantrums. Arch Gen Psychiatry 23:80–89, 1970

Malone RP, Biesecker KA, Delaney MA, et al: Youth self-report in aggression: baseline placebo responders and nonresponders, in Scientific Proceedings, American Academy of Child and Adolescent Psychiatry 41st Annual Meeting, New York, October 1994. New York, American Academy of Child and Adolescent Psychiatry, 1994a, p 49

Malone RP, Luebbert J, Pena-Ariet M, et al: The Overt Aggression Scale in a study of lithium in aggressive conduct disorder. Psychopharmacol Bull 30:215–218, 1994b

Malone RP, Delaney MA, Luebbert JF, et al: The lithium test dose prediction method in aggressive children. Psychopharmacol Bull 31: 379–382, 1995

Malone RP, Luebbert JF, Rowan AB, et al: Variables related to aggression during placebo baseline in conduct disorder. Poster presented at the 36th annual meeting of the New Clinical Drug Evaluation Program, National Institute of Mental Health, Boca Raton, FL, May 1996a

Malone RP, Rowan AB, Biesecker KA, et al: Aggression classification and treatment response. Poster presented at the 43rd annual meeting of the American Academy of Child and Adolescent Psychiatry, Philadelphia, PA, October 1996b

Malone RP, Rowan AB, Luebbert JF, et al: Lithium for the treatment of aggression in conduct disorder. Poster presented at the 43rd annual meeting of the American Academy of Child and Adolescent Psychiatry, Philadelphia, PA, October 1996c

McGuffin PW, Malone RP, Fergueson C, et al: The effect of lithium treatment for aggression on measures of cognition, in 1994 New Research Program and Abstracts, American Psychiatric Association Annual Meeting, Philadelphia, PA, May 21–26, 1994. Washington, DC, American Psychiatric Association, 1994, NR587, p 209

Molling PA, Lockner AW, Sauls RJ, et al: Committed delinquent boys. Arch Gen Psychiatry 7:96–102, 1962

Novaco RW: Anger as a risk factor for violence among the mentally disordered, in Violence and Mental Disorder: Developments in Risk Assessment. Edited by Monahan J, Steadman HJ. Chicago, IL, University of Chicago Press, 1994, pp 21–59

Palmstierna T, Wistedt B: Staff Observation Aggression Scale, SOAS: presentation and evaluation. Acta Psychiatr Scand 76:657–663, 1987

Perry R, Campbell M, Adams P, et al: Long-term efficacy of haloperidol in autistic children: continuous versus discontinuous drug administration. J Am Acad Child Adolesc Psychiatry 28:87–92, 1989

Pharmacotherapy of children. Psychopharmacol Bull (special issue) 1973

Platt JE, Campbell M, Green WH, et al: Cognitive effects of lithium carbonate and haloperidol in treatment-resistant aggressive children. Arch Gen Psychiatry 41:657–662, 1984

Puente RM: The use of carbamazepine in the treatment of behavioural disorders in children, in Epileptic Seizures–Behaviour–Pain. Edited by Birkmayer W. Bern, Switzerland, Hans Huber, 1976, pp 243–247

Rating scales and assessment instruments for use in pediatric psychopharmacology research (special issue). Psychopharmacol Bull 21(4), 1985

Rifkin A, Karajgi B, Perl E, et al: Lithium treatment of conduct disorders in adolescents. Paper presented at the 29th annual meeting of the New Clinical Drug Evaluation Program, National Institute of Mental Health, Key Biscayne, FL, June 1989

Robins LN: Deviant Children Grown Up: A Sociological and Psychiatric Study of Sociopathic Personality. Baltimore, MD, Williams & Wilkins, 1966

Robins LN: Longitudinal studies: sturdy childhood predictors of adult antisocial behaviour. Psychol Med 8:611–622, 1978

Safer DJ, Allen RP: Factors influencing the suppressant effects of two stimulant drugs on the growth of hyperactive children. Pediatrics 51:660–667, 1973

Safer D, Allen R, Barr E: Depression of growth in hyperactive children on stimulant drugs. N Engl J Med 287:217–220, 1972

Sheard MH: Effect of lithium on human aggression. Nature 230:113–114, 1971

Sheard MH: Lithium in the treatment of aggression. J Nerv Ment Dis 160:108–118, 1975

Sheard MH, Marini JL, Bridges CI, et al: The effect of lithium on impulsive aggressive behavior in man. Am J Psychiatry 133:1409–1413, 1976

Siever LJ, Coccaro EF, Trestman RL, et al: Use of serotonin-active agents in other psychiatric disorders. Clin Neuropharmacol 15 (suppl 1, pt A):355A–356A, 1992

Silva RR, Gonzalez NM, Kafantaris V, et al: Long-term use of lithium in aggressive conduct disordered children, in Scientific Proceedings, American Academy of Child and Adolescent Psychiatry 38th Annual Meeting, New York, October 1991. New York, American Academy of Child and Adolescent Psychiatry, 1991, p 74

Silva RR, Campbell M, Golden RR, et al: Side effects associated with lithium and placebo administration in aggressive children. Psychopharmacol Bull 28:319–326, 1992

Silver JM, Yudofsky SC: Documentation of aggression in the assessment of the violent patient. Psychiatric Annals 17:375–384, 1987

Sorgi P, Ratey JJ, Knoedler DW, et al: Rating aggression in the clinical setting: a retrospective adaptation of the Overt Aggression Scale. J Neuropsychiatry Clin Neurosci 3(suppl):S52–S56, 1991

Spielberger CD: Manual for the State-Trait Anger Expression Inventory (STAXI). Odessa, FL, Psychological Assessment Resources, 1988

Spielberger CD, Ritterband LM, Sydeman SJ, et al: Assessment of emotional states and personality traits: measuring psychological vital signs, in Clinical Personality Assessment: Practical Approaches. Edited by Butcher JN. New York, Oxford University Press, 1995, pp 42–58

Stewart MA: Aggressive conduct disorder: a brief review. Aggressive Behavior 11:323–331, 1985

Stewart M, Kelso J: A two-year follow-up of boys with aggressive conduct disorder. Psychopathology 20:296–304, 1987

Stoff DM, Pollock L, Vitiello B, et al: Reduction of (^{3}H)-imipramine binding sites on platelets of conduct-disordered children. Neuropsychopharmacology 1:55–62, 1987

Taylor SP: Aggressive behavior and physiological arousal as a function of provocation and the tendency to inhibit aggression. J Pers 35:297–310, 1967

U.S. Department of Health and Human Services: Healthy People 2000: National Health Promotion and Disease Prevention Objectives (DHHS Publ No PHS-91–50212). Washington, DC, U.S. Department of Health and Human Services, 1991

Vincent J, Varley CK, Leger P: Effects of methylphenidate on early adolescent growth. Am J Psychiatry 147:501–502, 1990

Vitiello B, Behar D, Hunt J, et al: Subtyping aggression in children and adolescents. J Neuropsychiatry Clin Neurosci 2:189–192, 1990

Werry JS, Wollersheim JP: Behavior therapy with children and adolescents: a twenty-year overview. J Am Acad Child Adolesc Psychiatry 28:1–18, 1989

Winsberg BG, Press M, Bialer I, et al: Dextroamphetamine and methylphenidate in the treatment of hyperactive-aggressive children. Pediatrics 53:236–241, 1974

Wistedt B, Rasmussen A, Pedersen L, et al: The development of an observer-scale for measuring social dysfunction and aggression. Pharmacopsychiatry 23:249–252, 1990

Yudofsky SC, Silver JM, Jackson W, et al: Overt Aggression Scale for objective rating of verbal and physical aggression. Am J Psychiatry 143:35–39, 1986

Zito JM, Riddle MA: Psychiatric pharmacoepidemiology for children. Child Adolesc Psychiatr Clin N Am 4:77–95, 1995

Zito JM, Craig TJ, Wanderling J: Pharmacoepidemiology of 330 child/adolescent psychiatric patients. Journal of Pharmacoepidemiology 3:47–62, 1994

CHAPTER 3

Managing Acutely Violent Inpatients

Laura Jane Bernay, M.D.
Devitt J. Elverson, M.D.

There is little in psychiatry that is more frightening than the threat of imminent violence. Violent patients pose a clear and immediate danger to other patients, staff, the therapeutic milieu, and themselves. Social initiatives such as deinstitutionalization, managed care, and severe limitation of psychiatric benefits have removed all but the very sickest patients from hospitals, leaving an inpatient population admitted or retained precisely because of dangerousness to self or others. A violent act is a complex behavior that is the culmination of a number of factors, both internal and external. It is the task of the inpatient psychiatrist and other members of the therapeutic team to recognize the signs of impending violence, to understand the reasons for violence, and to develop an armamentarium of techniques for the control of aggressive behavior.

In this chapter we discuss the evaluation and management of acutely violent adult inpatients. This chapter is divided into three sections. In the first section we briefly touch on the assessment of violent behavior, including diagnostic and psychosocial considerations. This topic is more fully discussed elsewhere in this volume (see Chapter 1). In the second section we discuss the management of imminent violence, including verbal interventions, medication management, and the use of restraint and seclusion. In the final section we briefly discuss the aftermath of violence, including debriefing and providing support for victimized staff and patients.

Evaluation of Acutely Violent Psychiatric Inpatients: General Considerations

Prevalence

Violent behavior is most likely to occur within the first few days after admission. At this point, patients may be incompletely evaluated and may not have begun treatment. Binder and McNiel (1990) found that 13.6% of men and 21.5% of women attacked another person within the first 3 days of hospitalization. The situation is quite different in chronic care facilities. Tardiff and Sweillam (1982) found that about 7% of long-term patients in both public and private facilities had an assault within the 3-month study period.

Psychopathology

Psychiatric diagnoses associated with violence range from psychotic disorders to mood disorders and from organic disorders such as delirium, dementia, and intoxication to personality disorders. Violent acts can occur as the result of the patient's response to a wide variety of psychopathology. A patient may experience command auditory hallucinations telling him or her to strike out. Patients experiencing visual hallucinations, such as those that occur in delirium tremens, may attempt to protect themselves from what they are seeing. Patients experiencing tactile hallucinations may become violent in an attempt to disengage themselves from whatever they are feeling. Under a delusional system a patient may perceive violence as his or her only option. Some patients become violent when they lose control over impulses, especially when these impulses are fueled by disturbances in affective state. Finally, the use of violence may be volitional or motivated by secondary gain.

It is helpful to understand the subjective experience of a patient in order to plan an empathic and helpful intervention. Understanding the patient's experience may provide the clinician with insight into what is fueling a violent episode and allow empathy. The affective states underlying and motivating violent behavior are most often fear, frustration, and anger. The experience of being understood and of being treated in a respectful manner will often help the patient respond without violence.

It is important to consider the violent patient's diagnosis in planning treatment, because the treatment of agitation in one diagnostic group may be contraindicated in a different group. A low-potency neuroleptic may be effective in the treatment of an agitated patient with schizophrenia, whereas it is contraindicated for a patient with delirium tremens because of its tendency to lower the seizure threshold. A benzodiazepine may calm an agitated patient with mania, but it may exacerbate agitation in a patient with dementia. A patient under the influence of a hallucinogen, such as PCP (phencyclidine hydrochloride), may respond to an environment where sensory stimulation is decreased, but decreased stimulation may cause a patient with dementia to become more agitated, a phenomenon commonly called *sundowning*.

Milieu

An environment in which the rules are clear, explicit, and consistent across shifts and for all patients can help decrease the likelihood of a violent episode. Forming a behavioral contract with a patient is often a very effective way of presenting explicit rules and engaging the patient in the treatment process. Contracts allow patients to feel that they have some input into, and thus responsibility for carrying out, a treatment plan. Agitated and assaultive patients are no exception. The patients' awareness that there are consequences, perhaps legal consequences, to an act of violence may help them gain control over violent impulses.

Cultural Issues

The concepts of respect and disrespect vary from culture to culture, as do acceptable boundaries of personal space. Perceptions of eye contact and of physical contact are very strongly culturally determined, as are gender-specific roles and ways of relating to members of the same and opposite sex. A patient's cultural background and values may often interact with other factors, such as diagnosis and milieu, to contribute to violent behavior. The clinician who is unaware of cultural variations may unwittingly commit a faux pas that offends or threatens a patient from a different cultural context.

Management

Verbal and Behavioral Techniques

The way in which staff interact with a patient may contribute to containing or exacerbating a violent episode. A calm, professional, confident approach to dealing with a patient whose aggressive behavior is escalating will often defuse a violent episode, whereas a hostile, threatening approach will usually be experienced as provocative and may be an impetus to violence. If, indeed, intimidation is successful in stemming a violent episode, it will usually be countertheraputic in the aftermath of such an episode and might interfere with the patient's ability to gain insight into his or her psychopathology.

"Talking Down"

An angry or agitated patient who has not yet lost control may be amenable to verbal interventions. However, patients who are profoundly impaired by psychosis, delirium, or cognitive deficits generally require immediate chemical or physical containment. As Soloff (1983) noted,

> The approach of "talking down" the potentially violent patient assumes that the patient can perceive the same causal reality as the clinician and, indeed, that verbal communication is meaningful at all. . . . While the psychodynamic philosophy has great appeal and efficacy in working with nonpsychotic or marginally psychotic (borderline) characters in crisis, its utility with decompensated psychotics must be tempered by the facts of the patient's actual behavior. . . . The occasional loss of life that has resulted from a physician's attempts to "talk down" violent patients serves as a stark reminder of our limited understanding of violence and the need to closely monitor behavior as the only reliable key to action. (p. 250)

Some patients, especially those with paranoid ideation, require less interpersonal stimulation, not more, in order to regain control. With these provisos in mind, verbal intervention may be a reasonable first step in the management of an agitated patient.

Isolation/Quiet Room

Most psychiatric wards have a room where a patient may go, voluntarily, with or without staff assistance, to be alone, away from frightening stimuli, or to experience painful affects. In some cases, the quiet room is simply the seclusion room with the door left ajar or the patient's own bedroom. Ideally, it would be a room where the patient can be comfortable, separate from other patients, but close to staff supervision. Allowing the patient to use the quiet room assumes that he or she is not immediately dangerous to himself or herself, or others.

Chemical Techniques

Agitated, potentially violent, or violent patients generally require rapid chemical control: medications with sedative and/or antipsychotic properties administered orally or parenterally. Neuroleptics and benzodiazepines are currently the mainstays of treatment of acute agitation.

In emergencies, medication may be administered without the patient's consent. When the patient's symptoms are ego-dystonic—that is, experienced as uncomfortable, abnormal, or frightening—the patient may ask for help in controlling them. Patients who have experienced relief from medication may ask for a prn medication before their symptoms escalate to dangerous levels.

Neuroleptics

There is much debate about which neuroleptic to select in treating an agitated patient. Many clinicians favor high-potency agents such as haloperidol, fluphenazine, thiothixene, or droperidol. These agents are less likely than low-potency agents to lower seizure threshold; have few, if any, cardiovascular side effects when administered orally or intramuscularly; and are generally viewed as safe and reliable. High-potency neuroleptics, when used alone, are only mildly sedating, especially in patients on chronic neuroleptic treatment. They are more likely than their lower-potency cousins to cause extrapyramidal side effects such as laryngospasm (which is potentially fatal), oculogyric crisis, and other acute dystonias. Akathisia—intense subjective restlessness—is far more common with high-potency neuroleptics and may be indistinguishable from worsening agitation.

Giving a sedative along with the high-potency neuroleptic solves many of these problems. Lorazepam is often coadministered with a neuroleptic because it provides additional sedation, protects against acute dystonias, and often ameliorates akathisia. Parenteral lorazepam is a viscous solution that cannot be combined with other drugs in the same syringe; therefore, combination therapy has the disadvantage of requiring two separate injections.

Low-potency neuroleptics have the advantage of being more sedating and more anticholinergic than high-potency neuroleptics. Thus, the physician has less concern about the occurrence of unwanted and potentially fatal side effects such as laryngospasm, dystonias, or other extrapyramidal effects. The use of a more sedating, low-potency neuroleptic may avert the need for an additional sedating or antiparkinsonian agent. However, the anticholinergic side effects of low-potency neuroleptics also carry a number of serious risks, including precipitation of anticholinergic delirium (characterized by dry, hot skin, dilated pupils, fever, tachycardia, and altered mental status), narrow-angle glaucoma, and urinary retention. Furthermore, the α-adrenergic properties of low-potency agents may result in orthostatic hypotension with tachycardia.

Neuroleptics are not a first-line treatment of agitation in a patient who is withdrawing from sedative-hypnotics or from alcohol, because these agents decrease the seizure threshold in patients already at risk of developing seizures. Neuroleptics, unlike benzodiazepines and barbiturates, are not cross-tolerant with alcohol or sedative-hypnotics and will not prevent delirium tremens or other life-threatening sequelae of withdrawal. Neuroleptics, particularly low-potency agents, should be used with caution, if at all, when deliriums of other etiologies are present. In this situation, determining the underlying cause of altered mental status is of critical importance. Low-dose haloperidol (or a similar high-potency neuroleptic) may be used for patient management during and after the evaluation period. In short, high-potency neuroleptics may be helpful in the management of some agitated states due to delirium, but they are not a treatment for delirium.

Rapid neuroleptization.   Until the mid-1980s, rapid neuroleptization was a common technique for the management of acutely psychotic patients, especially those who were violent or who were otherwise difficult to manage. Patients were given intramuscular (or sometimes intravenous) injections of a neuroleptic, generally a high-potency agent such as haloperidol, although some practitioners used low-potency neuroleptics, at a high frequency (e.g., every 1–2 hours), until the patient was sedated. In recent years, this technique has fallen out of favor and is no longer recommended. There is little theoretical justification for rapid administration of high-dose neuroleptic, insofar as dopamine receptors are thought to be saturated at relatively low doses of neuroleptic (e.g., 15 mg/day of haloperidol) (Wolkin et al. 1989). Empirical studies by Donlon et al. (1980) showed that rapid neuroleptization with doses of haloperidol up to 100 mg/day was no more effective in reducing symptoms than a standard fixed dose of 10 mg/day. High-dose strategies are associated with considerable morbidity, including dystonias (e.g., laryngospasm and oculogyric crisis, parkinsonian symptoms, and akathisia), which may exacerbate violence. Rapid intravenous neuroleptization is an even riskier procedure: there are reports of torsades de pointes, a dangerous ventricular arrhythmia, with intravenous haloperidol (Hunt and Stern 1995).

Alternatives to rapid neuroleptization: recommendations. In lieu of rapid neuroleptization, we recommend using a reasonable standing dose of a neuroleptic such as haloperidol 10–20 mg/day and then using prn medication consisting of a small dose of neuroleptic plus a sedative such as a benzodiazepine or a barbiturate every 6–8 hours as needed to maintain safety. Another reasonable alternative to rapid neuroleptization for agitated, psychotic patients is to switch the standing medication to a sedating neuroleptic such as chlorpromazine, thioridazine, or loxapine. This strategy is particularly good for patients with a history of sedative-hypnotic abuse (but not for those in acute withdrawal). If a prn medication is needed, chlorpromazine 25–50 mg intramuscularly (im) or loxapine 5 mg im can be given. Intramuscular doses of chlorpromazine should not exceed 50 mg except in rare cases of patients with extreme tolerance.

Benzodiazepines

Salzman et al. (1991) compared parenteral lorazepam with parenteral haloperidol for the emergency control of assaultive or aggressive behavior. Most of the patients in their study were already taking standing neuroleptic medication. Patients requiring prn medication were given either haloperidol 5 mg im or lorazepam 2 mg im in a double-blind fashion. Patients were rated on the Overt Aggression Scale (OAS; Yudofsky et al. 1986) and the Brief Psychiatric Rating Scale (BPRS; Guy 1976); side effects and sedation were also rated. The investigators found that both groups had a significant reduction in aggressivity as measured by the OAS and psychosis as measured by the BPRS. The two agents appeared to be equally sedating insofar as about one-third of the patients in each group fell asleep within 1 hour after receiving their injection. On the other hand, patients receiving haloperidol were 11 times more likely than lorazepam recipients to have extrapyramidal side effects such as akathisia and dystonia. Salzman et al. concluded that parenteral lorazepam is as effective as parenteral haloperidol in the acute management of aggressive behavior, produces fewer side effects than haloperidol, and may be safer than haloperidol.

Midazolam is a highly lipophilic benzodiazepine marketed as a preanesthetic agent because of its rapid onset of sedation. Sedation begins 5–15 minutes after intramuscular administration and peaks at 30–60 minutes after administration. Midazolam is rapidly cleared and thus has a very short duration of action: about 2 hours, with a range of 1 to 6 hours. The incidence of respiratory depression is relatively low when midazolam is administered intramuscularly. Although no double-blind studies have been reported, there are several case reports of midazolam successfully calming acutely agitated or violent psychiatric patients very rapidly (Bond et al. 1989).

It is important to remember that no other benzodiazepines currently available are absorbed intramuscularly. Therefore, agents such as diazepam should never be used via the intramuscular route.

Barbiturates

Until the advent of reliably absorbed forms of parenteral benzodiazepines, barbiturates were a common alternative to parenteral neuroleptics. Their use is still valid and preferred by some practitioners for the treatment of acutely agitated patients. They are especially useful in the treatment of patients with serious adverse reactions to benzodiazepines or those in whom benzodiazepines are ineffective. Barbiturates with half-lives in the range of 15–40 hours are preferable to barbiturates with longer half-lives because of the risks of accumulation of longer-acting drugs.

The most commonly used barbiturate for the treatment of agitation is amobarbital. In general, the adverse effects of barbiturates are similar to those found with benzodiazepines: dysphoria, paradoxical hyperactivity, and cognitive disorganization. Barbiturates have a high potential for abuse, tolerance, and dependence, and a low therapeutic index. Barbiturates can precipitate crisis in patients with previously unrecognized acute intermittent porphyria.

Pharmacological Management of the Elderly and Medically Ill: Special Considerations

Elderly patients are especially sensitive to the side effects of psychotropic drugs. Neuroleptics, especially low-potency agents such as chlorpromazine, can induce orthostatic hypotension, which may result in falls and fractures. Elderly patients may become oversedated or confused by low-potency agents. They are also highly susceptible to the extrapyramidal side effects of neuroleptics; dystonias, parkinsonian symptoms, and akathisia can occur in elderly patients treated with any neuroleptic, but the high-potency agents, such as haloperidol or fluphenazine, are most likely to result in these side effects. Elderly patients who are treated with antipsychotic agents are also at risk for neuroleptic malignant syndrome, which presents with high fevers, lead pipe rigidity, elevated creatine phosphokinase levels, and altered mental status. Benzodiazepines and other sedative-hypnotic drugs are also problematic in the elderly because, like low-potency neuroleptics, they may result in oversedation or confusion. Other risks with benzodiazepines include mood disturbances, especially dysphoria, worsening cognitive functioning, paradoxical excitement, and behavioral disinhibition.

The treatment approach with aggressive elderly patients depends on their history. Elderly patients with a long history of psychiatric illness and treatment with psychotropic agents will be able to tolerate higher doses of medication than an elderly patient with new-onset psychiatric symptoms who has never received psychotropic drugs. The old saw to "start low and go slow" for geriatric patients holds true even in the treatment of agitation or violence. Acute management of agitation in the elderly is generally accomplished with low-dose haloperidol or lorazepam, or a combination of the two, administered orally or intramuscularly. For elderly or debilitated patients, haloperidol oral concentrate 1 mg or haloperidol 0.5 mg im may be given once an hour until the behavior is controlled. Alternatively, lorazepam 1 mg may be given orally or intramuscularly, alone or in combination with haloperidol. A third choice might be very-low-dose chlorpromazine, which has the advantage of having both antipsychotic and sedating effects, although patients with underlying central nervous system impairment may be exquisitely sensitive to anticholinergic side effects.

Physical Techniques: Seclusion and Restraint

Much of contemporary psychiatry is governed by the principle of the *least restrictive alternative*. Thus, we often view the use of physical techniques as the treatment of last resort and feel that they represent the failure of previous therapeutic efforts. Patients generally prefer medication or verbal interventions over seclusion or restraint; most experience physical interventions as traumatic, dehumanizing, or humiliating. Seclusion and restraint can be high-risk activities for staff, too. In one study, 86 of 135 staff injuries in a forensic hospital and 15 of 46 staff injuries at a state hospital occurred during administration of seclusion or restraint (Fisher 1994).

Nonetheless, physical containment techniques are effective and often necessary on inpatient wards. Gerlock and Solomons (1983) found that whereas 83% of patients showed disturbed behavior prior to being secluded, only 23% showed disturbed behavior when released. Physical containment techniques are often required because pharmacological and psychosocial treatments for the underlying causes of violence may not work rapidly enough to protect patients, personnel, and the environment. Certain violent patients, especially antisocial patients with directed, instrumental violence, are not highly responsive to pharmacotherapy.

The purpose of physical techniques is to contain dangerous impulses or to protect the patient from perceptual or interpersonal overstimulation when the patient's internal controls are inadequate. Psychiatrists working in an inpatient environment should be comfortable with seclusion and restraint procedures and familiar with local regulations regarding their use. Seclusion and/or restraint is a relatively common experience for psychiatric patients. Soloff and Turner (1981), in a prospective study, found that 10.5% of all admitted patients required a physical intervention at least once during their 8-month study period.

Patients almost always experience seclusion or restraint as aversive, and for many it is traumatic. Patients may become fearful, angry, paranoid, or guilty; some experience worsened hallucinations, possibly in response to sensory deprivation. Binder and McCoy (1983) studied patients' attitudes toward seclusion and found that 13 of 24 had no idea or a false idea about why they had been placed in seclusion. When asked about the experience, half the patients said they thought it had been necessary and would not adversely affect their attitudes toward treatment. Other patients complained that seclusion made them feel humiliated, lonely, or trapped.

Indications and Contraindications

In 1984, the American Psychiatric Association Task Force on Seclusion and Restraint (American Psychiatric Association 1985, p. 17) enumerated the indications for the use of physical techniques:

- *"To prevent imminent harm to the patient or other persons when other means of control are not effective or appropriate."* For example, a patient who is making direct verbal or physical threats to a specific person and who cannot be dissuaded from pursuing the victim, or a patient who is wielding a weapon or an ordinary object that might be used as a weapon or projectile in a threatening manner, or a suicidal or self-mutilating patient who cannot be deterred from self-harm, or a patient threatening sexual assault.

- *"To prevent serious disruption of the treatment program ..."* For example, an agitated, angry, and hyperactive patient who prevents others from participating in therapeutic activities, or a profoundly regressed psychotic patient demonstrating primitive behaviors such as smearing feces, or a patient engaged in public masturbation, or a patient who is verbally harassing staff or peers engaged in a therapeutic group. Using seclusion or restraint in defense of the milieu can be justified only if it is also an appropriate therapeutic intervention for the patient's psychiatric condition. For example, it would not be appropriate to use seclusion if the patient disrupting the environment was experiencing delirium tremens or catatonic excitement.
- *"To prevent . . . significant damage to the physical environment."* For example, a patient who is smashing furniture, breaking down doors, setting fires, or destroying other patients' personal property.
- *"For treatment as part of an ongoing plan of behavior therapy."* As a contingency in the behavior therapy of dangerous behaviors. For example, a chronically assaultive patient who has agreed to a behavioral contract in which any explicit threats against others will result in placement in seclusion or restraint.
- *"To decrease the stimulation a patient receives."* For example, an acutely psychotic patient with paranoid schizophrenia who is profoundly frightened by the presence of other people, or a severely manic patient already overstimulated and exhausted because of internal stimuli.
- *"Use at the request of a patient."* For example, a patient who retains insight despite loss of impulse control requesting physical separation in order to prevent himself or herself from harming others.

In actual clinical practice, seclusion and restraint are most often used to prevent violence. Nonviolent behaviors are more common precipitants to physical intervention than actual violence. The most common reason given for secluding or restraining patients is "behavior disruptive to the therapeutic environment" (Soloff et al. 1985).

Way and Banks (1990) studied seclusion and restraint in 23 New York State psychiatric hospitals over a 1-month period. They found that 657 patients were involved in 1,409 episodes of seclusion or restraint. Overall, across hospitals, 2.8% of patients were placed in seclusion or restraint, with the proportion of patients secluded or restrained ranging from 0.4% to 9.4%. Secluded patients tended to be younger, with a median age of 31 years, as compared with nonsecluded patients, who had a median age of 58 years. In the chronic care facilities where this study was performed, the highest probability of being secluded or restrained was within the first 30 to 365 days of hospitalization. Way and Banks found that males were more likely to be secluded or restrained than females. Race bore no relationship to rates of seclusion and restraint. In acute care settings patients carrying a diagnosis of schizophrenia or mania are most likely to undergo seclusion or restraint, whereas in chronic care settings, patients with mental retardation and nonpsychotic patients have the highest rates (Soloff et al. 1985).

In a review of seclusion and restraint, Fisher (1994) compiled a list of *contraindications.* Seclusion and restraint should *not* be used

- With patients with encephalopathy, which can be exacerbated by decreased sensory input
- As a substitute for treatment
- As a punishment
- As a response to obnoxious behavior
- For staff convenience
- When experienced by the patient as a positive reinforcement for violence
- With patients who are medically unstable

In addition to these contraindications, we would add that *seclusion should never be used for self-mutilative or imminently suicidal patients,* although restraints may safely be used in these circumstances. The psychiatrist should be aware of local statutes and regulations; for example, about 50% of states do not permit the use of physical techniques as a contingency in behavior therapy; New York State does not permit seclusion of mentally retarded persons. In addition, there may be site-specific rules based on institutional policy or philosophy governing the use of these techniques.

Procedure

Physical containment of a patient may be initiated and carried out by any member of the clinical staff, but is most often the responsibility of nursing staff. Ideally, a team is deployed of at least five staff members who have been trained in procedures of seclusion and restraint and who have worked and trained together. One person is designated the leader; this person directs all of the action until the patient is safely contained. The leader should be someone well trained in these techniques who has a therapeutic alliance with the patient and a working relationship with the staff. The leader does not have to be physically powerful; in fact, patients sometimes respond better to smaller, less-imposing staff members. Once the seclusion or restraint procedure has begun, all communication with the patient must be through the leader. Otherwise, the patient may receive mixed or ambiguous messages from the staff and may attempt to split the staff, resulting in a more chaotic and dangerous situation. When the seclusion leader is a therapy aide, professional staff must take a secondary role, as difficult as it may be for them to do so.

The leader assigns roles to the other members of the team: one person is assigned to each extremity and one person to control the head. If there is sufficient personnel, a sixth person is assigned to monitoring and documenting the proceedings and to debriefing and critiquing the staff afterward. If possible, other staff members may be called on, to make an adequate "show of force." They may also be needed to remove other patients from the vicinity and to supervise them while the containment is being done.

During the preparatory period, team members should remove their jewelry, pagers, keys, and, if practicable, eyeglasses, as well as anything else on their person that could be grabbed by the patient or be used as a weapon. Universal infection control precautions should be observed; those personnel who will have hands-on contact with the patient should wear latex gloves. If medication is to be administered, a nurse should begin preparing it as soon as the decision is made to intervene.

The team approaches, and the leader tells the patient that his or her behavior is dangerous and must be contained. The patient is told that he or she will be secluded or restrained and is given the option of walking with the staff to the seclusion room. The patient may be given a minute or two to decide to go into seclusion or restraint willingly. It is important to remember that once the patient's behavior has escalated to assaultiveness or extremely destructive or dangerous behavior, the time for psychodynamic interpretations or behavioral contract negotiation has passed.

If a very clear message has been conveyed to the patient that containment is not negotiable at this stage, the patient may opt to go willingly, because this is less physically threatening and less humiliating than being forcibly brought down. If the patient is willing, the staff should surround the patient, with the team members assigned to upper extremities gently but firmly grasping the patient's upper arms and leading the way to the seclusion room.

If the patient refuses to cooperate, the leader signals the team to begin. One staff member secures each extremity, taking care to protect the joints. Another staff member, standing behind the patient, controls the head, preventing it from hitting the ground when the patient is taken down and preventing the patient from biting staff. The staff member assigned to the head is also responsible for monitoring the patient's neck and airway. This is a crucial job; patient deaths during seclusion and restraint have occurred because of airway obstruction. At the leader's signal, the patient's legs are raised while the upper body and head are gently lowered to the floor. Then the whole body is lowered, horizontally, to the floor. The head and each extremity are secured by the assigned personnel, and the patient is carried in the supine position, feet first, to the seclusion room. Care should be taken that the proximal and distal ends of the extremities are secured, both to protect the patient's joints and to prevent the patient from using arms or legs to injure the staff.

Once in the seclusion room, the patient is placed on a mattress in the supine position, with the head closest to the door. Intramuscular medication, if indicated, should be administered at this time, using either the deltoid or gluteus muscle as the injection site. Absorption of medication is somewhat superior from the deltoid, but patients may resist attempts to completely immobilize the arm, which can put staff at risk for needle-stick injuries. If the gluteus is chosen, the team may roll the patient onto his or her side and draw aside any clothing covering the buttock.

If the patient is to be secluded, the staff must remove all potentially dangerous objects. Such items include, but are not limited to, shoes, belts, jewelry, eyeglasses, writing implements, and cutlery. Some hospitals require that patients be secluded in a hospital gown, whereas others allow patients to be secluded in their own clothing as long as it is safe. If possible, the patient's vital signs should be checked and recorded, although in actual practice this is frequently very difficult to achieve.

The staff should leave the seclusion room one at a time according to a prearranged plan. The personnel managing the lower extremities leave first, then those controlling the upper extremities, and finally the person at the patient's head, who backs out of the seclusion room and closes the door behind himself or herself.

A seclusion room, according to the APA Task Force (American Psychiatric Association 1985), should have smooth walls, no furniture except a mattress, adequate lighting, and adequate climate control. In addition, the door must be secured by a deadbolt so that the inhabitant cannot voluntarily egress nor be released by a casual passerby (e.g., a well-meaning patient). There must be an observation window made from Lexan, Plexiglas, or other nonshattering material. Light bulbs should be protected by wire mesh. Climate control equipment must be inaccessible to the patient.

If the patient is to be restrained rather than secluded, the procedure is similar. The patient is placed on the bed in the supine position and restraints are applied to the extremities, with care taken that they are secure enough to contain the patient but not so tight as to compromise circulation. In some cases, a chest restraint may also be necessary to completely restrain an extremely agitated patient. We advise against the practice of restraining the patient on a gurney; a large, violently thrashing patient can overturn the gurney and can sustain serious injuries.

Authorization and Documentation

Seclusion or restraint is usually initiated by the nursing staff. The APA Task Force (American Psychiatric Association 1985) recommends that medical authorization be obtained within 1 hour after initiating the procedure. Most jurisdictions require a personal examination by a physician within 1–12 hours, as well as a nursing examination, including level of consciousness, vital signs (temperature, pulse, respiration, and blood pressure), and hydration. A physician's order for physical containment is valid for a variable period of time, 1–24 hours, depending on state law. Orders for physical containment should, at minimum, contain the following:

- Date and time the order was written
- Type of containment
- Exact times for which the order is valid
- Reason for containment
- Criteria for release
- Physician's signature and printed, or stamped, name

In addition, the physician should make a note in the patient's chart that includes the following information:

- Time the physician was informed of the physical intervention and the time the physician examined the patient
- Staff reports or personal observations of the problematic behavior
- A brief mental status examination
- Patient's physical condition, including presence of current medical conditions and indication of special medical requirements
- Description of results of less restrictive procedures tried prior to restraining the patient
- Medication(s) administered to the patient, including dose, route, and response

- Rationale for use of physical controls (e.g., dangerousness to self or others)
- Criteria for release

Supervision of the Secluded/Restrained Patient

Once the patient is in seclusion or restraint, the APA Task Force recommends reevaluation by the responsible physician at least twice a day. It further recommends that orders for physical containment remain valid for no more than 12 hours. Nursing staff should observe the patient every 15 minutes, speak with the patient at least every 2 hours, and attend to toilet needs at least every 4 hours. Patients in four-point restraints should have the circulation in their extremities checked every 15 minutes. Patients should receive meals as well as fluids; intake and output should be documented on the observation sheet. Finally, the APA Task Force recommends that after 72 hours of continuous seclusion or restraint the approval of the hospital director, or the director's designee, be obtained.

Duration of Containment

A number of studies have shown that there is little relation between the length of time a patient spends in seclusion or restraint and a number of variables, including the nature of the precipitant, diagnosis, or patient demographics. Soloff and Turner (1981) found a mean duration of 10.8 hours, a median of 2.8 hours, and a range of 10 minutes to 120 hours. Duration of containment should depend primarily on the patient's condition but also on the ward atmosphere. To release a marginally controlled patient into a volatile environment is potentially dangerous. Overall, we believe that, given the aversive nature of seclusion and restraint, patients should be released, at least for a trial period, as soon as they demonstrate that they can control their behavior.

Choosing a Method of Containment

Various methods of containment may be available to the treatment team, depending on local regulations and custom, including camisole, four- and five-point restraints, body blankets, cold wetpacks, and belt-to-wrist restraint. When physical containment is required, the choice of technique should be individualized to meet the needs of the patient, staff, and milieu. Some patients may benefit from the radically reduced perceptual and social stimulation provided by the isolation room. It should be kept in mind, however, that long periods of sensory deprivation can cause perceptual disturbances even in psychiatrically healthy subjects. Some patients may have exacerbation of psychotic symptoms, especially increased hallucinatory behavior, in the seclusion room. We have also seen a few patients who had severe psychotic regression to primitive behavior, such as soiling and smearing feces, in seclusion. A suicidal patient may find means of harming himself or herself in the seclusion room; for example, a patient removed the mattress ticking and attempted to garrote himself. Patients who remain capable of verbal communication despite loss of impulse control may benefit from mechanical restraint so that the clinician can maintain therapeutic involvement with the patient without fear of injury.

Aftermath of Violence

Debriefing

After a violent event, it is important for the treatment team to sit down together to review what happened before the event, what measures they took to calm the patient and ensure safety, and whether the patient's treatment plan requires revisions and, if so, how the revisions will be implemented. This review can minimize the risk of recurrent violence.

It is helpful to identify the precipitants that led to a violent act or behaviors that signaled that the patient was beginning to escalate his or her aggressive behavior. Could the violence have been predicted or prevented? Identifying precipitating events can help the perpetrator learn nonviolent means of coping with stressors or provocations.

It is also useful to review staff attempts to de-escalate the patient's aggressive behavior prior to the violent episode. Was there a team approach with a clearly identified leader? Was the patient treated with respect? Was there something about the way staff approached the patient that could have led the patient to escalate his or her behavior? Would the patient have responded differently to someone else, a staff member of the same gender or from a similar cultural background? If the patient was secluded or restrained, was this done in a way that minimized risk of injury to patient and staff?

The patient's medication regimen and compliance should be reexamined. If the patient has required frequent administrations of additional, as needed, medication, the dose or type of standing medication may need to be changed. If poor compliance is suspected, it may be necessary to switch to a liquid preparation.

Support for Victimized Staff and Patients

Staff or patients who have been the victim of an assault also need attention. Whether or not the assault has resulted in physical injury, there may be psychological sequelae such as rage, a wish for revenge, depression, fear, or posttraumatic stress disorder. Unfortunately, on short-staffed, overcrowded wards, the victim is often forgotten in the flurry of activity to contain the perpetrator. After attending to the victim's immediate medical needs, his or her psychological needs must also be considered. Victimized patients should be given the opportunity to talk over the incident with staff and with their primary therapist as soon after the event as possible. If the assault has been against more than one patient, or against the environment or therapeutic milieu, an emergency community meeting can be held to give all the patients an opportunity to express their thoughts and feelings.

Witnessing violence is traumatic and frightening; patients need the support of the staff in the hours after a serious incident. Staff who have been victimized may also need support and sometimes counseling. Flannery et al. (1991) found that a voluntary approach worked best: staff victims of assault were approached by a clinician from any of the departments of nursing, psychiatry, psychology, or social work immediately after the assault. The clinician assessed the victim's ability to return to work, ability to manage painful affects, support system, and understanding of the incident. The clinician also made a preliminary assessment for the presence of posttraumatic stress disorder. The victim was offered on-site counseling, a short-term support group for victims of assault, and/or referral to outside psychotherapy. Participation in any of these services was voluntary.

Conclusion

Understanding and managing violent patients is a clinical challenge for both new and seasoned psychiatrists. Overcoming one's own fear is often the first step in empathic treatment of these very difficult patients. Accurate diagnostic evaluation can uncover specific causes of violent behavior and guide treatment planning. Gaining mastery over psychosocial interventions, psychopharmacological agents, and physical techniques will make the task of treating these difficult-to-manage patients less daunting. Ultimately, helping violent patients bring their dangerous impulses under control can be one of psychiatry's greatest rewards.

References

American Psychiatric Association: Seclusion and Restraint: The Psychiatric Uses (Task Force Report 22). Washington, DC, American Psychiatric Association, 1985

Binder RL, McCoy SM: A study of patients' attitudes toward placement in seclusion. Hospital and Community Psychiatry 34:1052–1054, 1983

Binder RL, McNiel DE: The relationship of gender to violent behavior in acutely disturbed psychiatric patients. J Clin Psychiatry 51:110–114, 1990

Bond WS, Mandos LA, Kurtz MB: Midazolam for aggressivity and violence in three mentally retarded patients. Am J Psychiatry 146:925–926, 1989

Donlon PT, Hopkin JT, Tupin JP, et al: Haloperidol for acute schizophrenic patients: an evaluation of three oral regimens. Arch Gen Psychiatry 37:691–695, 1980

Fisher WA: Restraint and seclusion: a review of the literature. Am J Psychiatry 151:1584–1591, 1994

Flannery RB, Fulton F, Tausch J, et al: A program to help staff cope with psychological sequelae of assaults by patients. Hospital and Community Psychiatry 42:935–938, 1991

Gerlock A, Solomons HC: Factors associated with the seclusion of psychiatric patients. Perspectives on Psychiatric Care 21:46–53, 1983

Guy W: ECDEU Assessment Manual for Psychopharmacology—Revised (DHEW Publ No ADM-76–338). Rockville, MD, U.S. Department of Health, Education and Welfare, 1976

Hunt N, Stern TA: The association between intravenous haloperidol and torsades de pointes: three cases and a literature review. Psychosomatics 36:544–549, 1995

Salzman C, Solomon D, Miyawaki E, et al: Parenteral lorazepam versus parenteral haloperidol for the control of psychotic disruptive behavior. J Clin Psychiatry 52:177–180, 1991

Soloff PH: Seclusion and restraint, in Assaults Within Psychiatric Facilities. Edited by Lion JR, Reid WH. New York, Grune & Stratton, 1983, pp 241–264

Soloff PH, Turner SM: Patterns of seclusion: a prospective study. J Nerv Ment Dis 169:37–44, 1981

Soloff PH, Gutheil TG, Wexler DB: Seclusion and restraint in 1985: a review and update. Hospital and Community Psychiatry 36:652–657, 1985

Tardiff K, Sweillam A: Assaultive behavior among chronic inpatients. Am J Psychiatry 139:212–215, 1982

Way BB, Banks SM: Use of seclusion and restraint in public psychiatric hospitals: patient characteristics and facility effects. Hospital and Community Psychiatry 41:75–81, 1990

Wolkin A, Brodie J, Barouch F, et al: Dopamine receptor occupancy and plasma haloperidol levels. Arch Gen Psychiatry 46:482–484, 1989

Yudofsky SC, Silver JM, Jackson W, et al: The Overt Aggression Scale for the objective rating of verbal and physical aggression. Am J Psychiatry 143:35–39, 1986

CHAPTER 4

Behavior Therapy for Aggressive Psychiatric Patients

Patrick W. Corrigan, Psy.D.
Kim T. Mueser, Ph.D.

___

The aggressive behaviors of psychiatric patients may be caused by biological factors or environmental contingencies, or by interactions between them. Treatment teams are best prepared to deal with these behaviors when they draw from an armamentarium that includes interventions that address both biological and environmental factors. Psychopharmacological interventions are well suited for the biological precursors of aggression. Behavioral strategies—the focus of this chapter—are useful for managing types of aggression that have environmental antecedents or represent an interaction of biological and environmental factors.

The complex interaction of biological and environmental factors is well described by stress vulnerability models of mental illness. Such models not only suggest how biological and environmental factors may cause psychotic symptoms and interpersonal dysfunctions, but also suggest appropriate directions for intervention. A stress vulnerability model is used in this chapter to identify factors that may explain aggressive behavior and to identify strategies that will remediate these factors.

We begin this chapter with a review of the vulnerability model and how its components may predict aggression. We then review behavioral strategies that address these components. Specific strategies include behavior family therapy, social and coping skills training, and a range of behavioral interventions that decelerate violence. The token economy is briefly reviewed here and more thoroughly discussed by Dr. Menditto and colleagues in this volume (see Chapter 5).

Psychiatric Illness as Stress Vulnerability

Research suggests that the complex pattern of psychotic symptoms and social dysfunction common to most severe mental illnesses is the result of certain stress vulnerabilities (Nuechterlein et al. 1992); one version of the stress vulnerability model is summarized in Figure 4–1. According to this model, biological vulnerabilities interact with environmental stressors to cause psychiatric symptoms. It is still not clear whether these biological vulnerabilities occur because of genetic factors, in utero insults, or early childhood pathogens (Torrey et al. 1994). Research suggests, however, that these vulnerabilities are present during childhood and emerge as subtle deficits in cognition and modulation of psychophysiological arousal (Asarnow et al. 1994).

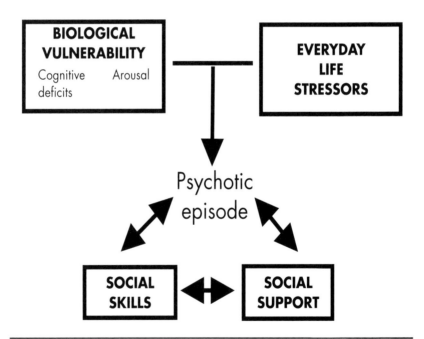

Figure 4–1.   *Interaction of biological vulnerabilities and environmental factors that account for psychiatric symptoms.* Note that specific agents seem to exacerbate aggressive behaviors.

Adults with severe mental illness have difficulty learning skills and building social support. Positive symptoms in particular can be so distracting that patients cannot attend to and vicariously learn the subtleties of interpersonal behavior, with the result that their ability to acquire social and coping skills is impaired (Lukoff et al. 1992). Cognitive deficits in the domains of attention and memory also hinder the ability of schizophrenic patients to learn fundamental social and coping skills (Spaulding et al. 1996). Patients may be unable to sustain attention to social situations and so are less likely to fully appreciate all aspects of a problem. Memory deficits can limit understanding of complex interpersonal situations. Individuals with deficient social skills tend to alienate family members and friends. Therefore, those most in need of interpersonal buffers to everyday stressors lack the social support that might best help them.

Social skills and social support are especially necessary for severely ill patients because they tend to be tonically hyperaroused. Any additional arousal, such as that engendered by everyday stress, can be intolerable for them. Eventually, life stressors combine with relatively enduring vulnerabilities to cause prodromal symptoms and, later on, an acute psychotic episode.

The stress vulnerability model suggests putative factors that may cause or exacerbate aggression in psychiatric patients. These factors, in turn, suggest behavioral strategies that might diminish hostility and aggression. Four elements of the model, highlighted in Figure 4–1, are particularly relevant. First, overarousal may increase the likelihood of hostility and aggression. Individuals who are psychophysiologically aroused because of social anxiety, worry, lack of sleep, or the influence of drugs are more easily frustrated by everyday problems (Bushman and Cooper 1990). This frustration can lead to angry responses and aggression. (For example, Frank was snapping more at his secretary about typing mistakes because he had not been sleeping well the past few nights.) Patients who are typically hyperaroused are likely to have a lower threshold for anger. Therefore, interventions that help to moderate patients' arousal or diminish environmental frustrations may diminish aggression. Behavioral strategies help patients to address factors in the social milieu that contribute to or maintain high levels of arousal.

Second, cognitive deficits greatly diminish an individual's ability to interact with others in nonaggressive, socially acceptable ways. Deficits in attention and memory may prevent them from accurately understanding interpersonal situations that give rise to frustration and dilemma. This problem is compounded in individuals with severe mental illness who are not able to sustain attention to social situations; as a result, they are less likely to fully comprehend all aspects of a problem. Therefore, strategies that seek to remedy the social deficits of severe mental illness must include interventions that diminish the learning disabilities brought on by primary cognitive impairments. In this chapter we describe one approach to this problem: a training program for cognitive skills.

Third, social skills deficits can make it difficult for the individual to resolve interpersonal problems appropriately without resorting to undue anger or aggression. Interpersonal problems are less likely to lead to aggression when the individual has a broad repertoire of social skills. (For example, Sarah was able to keep from fighting with a pushy sales-lady by asserting that she did not need her service.) Skills training strategies help patients to learn a variety of social and coping skills that are appropriate for resolving interpersonal difficulties.

Finally, lack of or deficient social support can contribute to an individual's being unable to deal with frustrations when faced with interpersonal conflict. Individuals with satisfactory social support may be able to resolve some of their frustrations with the help of this support system rather than becoming angry during interpersonal distress. (For example, Martha discussed her angry feelings about her boss with her husband, thereby defusing an unpleasant encounter with the employer.) Improved social skills frequently lead to broader and more satisfactory social support.

Overarousal, cognitive deficit, lack of social skills, and deficient social support are all factors that may cause or exacerbate aggression in psychiatric patients. In the remainder of this chapter we describe behavioral strategies that diminish the impact of overarousal and social skills deficits and help patients find alternatives to aggression. We also describe intervention strategies for disruptive and aggressive behavior.

Behavioral Strategies for Factors in Aggression

Overarousal

Several strategies can be used to decrease the effects of psychophysiological arousal on aggression. In particular, behavioral strategies address environmental factors within the social milieu that may contribute to or maintain overarousal.

Milieu-based methods are predicated on the assumption that environmental conditions, such as tense, hostile, chaotic, or conflict-ridden environments, can increase psychophysiological arousal and, hence, susceptibility to aggression. Modifying environmental contingencies that maintain negative behaviors, which in turn lead to high levels of arousal, and teaching alternative skills for managing conflict with others in the patient's environment may reduce arousal. Two of the most commonly used social-learning interventions that focus on the milieu are the token economy and behavioral family therapy.

Token Economy

The token economy is an operant behavioral approach to modifying patient behavior through the direct manipulation of contingencies under which patients operate (Corrigan 1995). Contingencies are if-then relationships between targeted behaviors and consequent rewards. For example, a patient may be informed that "if you brush your teeth each morning, then I will let you watch TV an extra hour." A related way to increase specific target behaviors is to give patients "tokens" rather than primary rewards (e.g., food or a chance to watch TV) for engaging in behaviors. (For example, Fred received five tokens for getting out of bed on time and Mary received two tokens for attending therapy group.) These tokens can then be exchanged for reinforcers valued by the patient. Undesirable behaviors may be decreased by attaching a "response cost" to the behavior (e.g., fining the patient tokens) or limiting access to potential reinforcers (e.g., time-out). A patient may be informed, "If you yell loudly, I will take away 10 tokens." Rigorous research on the token economy has demonstrated that it is effective at reducing violent behavior in psychiatric inpatients (Paul and Lentz 1977). The token-economy approach is discussed more fully in the chapter by Menditto and colleagues in this volume (see Chapter 5).

Behavioral Family Therapy

An alternative approach to the token economy for patients who reside with or have frequent contact with relatives is behavioral family therapy (Falloon et al. 1985; Mueser and Glynn 1995). Family interventions are important for psychiatric patients in contact with relatives because relatives are often the object of patient aggression (Estroff et al. 1994; Straznickas et al. 1993; Tardiff 1984). Furthermore, aggression in families with a psychiatric patient is often reciprocal, with both patients and relatives playing active roles in perpetuating aggression (Cascardi et al. 1996). Behavioral family therapy is one fruitful strategy for improving the family's ability to manage conflict effectively.

The goals of behavioral family therapy are to educate the family, to involve them in the patient's treatment, and to provide skills. Family therapists teach family members about the patient's illness, including its symptoms and treatment. Therapists promote more realistic expectations for the patient's behavior, given the extent of his or her disability. Family members are taught to monitor the course of the psychiatric illness and to foster gradual improvement. They are also taught to detect early signs of impending relapse and to reinforce gradual improvements toward self-management and self-sufficiency. Therapists then provide a structured program of communication and problem-solving skills training.

Behavioral family therapy can be effective in reducing aggressive behavior in psychiatric patients in three ways. First, it can reduce stress, and hence arousal, in the whole family and so decrease the likelihood of stress-induced relapses and aggression related to relapse. Second, it can improve the collective ability of the family to monitor the course of the psychiatric illness and so enable them to detect early warning signs of relapse, such as agitation, before a relapse occurs. Early detection and intervention during the prodrome of a relapse can avert full-blown relapses and attendant aggression (Birchwood et al. 1989). Third, by enhancing the ability of family members to successfully resolve conflict, behavioral family therapy can reduce aggressive episodes that stem from frustrating, unresolved conflicts between family members.

Behavioral family therapy is usually provided to individual families, including the patient, in therapy sessions lasting approximately 1 hour. Sessions are conducted for a year or more, with gradually declining contact over successive months. The focus of the sessions is on teaching new information and interpersonal skills, as well as providing support to family members, rather than fostering "insight" or delving into the past. Sessions may be conducted either at the home or the clinic, or at both. As outlined in Table 4–1, behavioral family therapy is often divided into five phases.

Table 4–1.   The five phases of behavioral family therapy

Assessment

Education about the psychiatric disorder

Communication skills training

Problem-solving training

Additional strategies for unresolved problems

During the *assessment phase,* the clinician meets individually with each family member to determine his or her understanding of the patient's illness and personal goals for therapy. Information gathered from individual interviews is supplemented by naturalistic observations of the family's strengths and weaknesses in communication and problem-solving skills. Assessments are repeated every 3–6 months throughout the course of therapy to determine progress toward personal goals.

Following the assessment phase, *educational sessions* are devoted to informing family members about the characteristic symptoms of the disorder, the pharmacological treatments and their side effects, and the role family members can play in its management. Educational sessions are highly interactive, aimed at eliciting experiences with the illness of both the patient and his or her relatives.

When a basic understanding of the nature of the psychiatric illness and of the principles of its treatment has been established over the course of the educational sessions, the next step in behavioral family therapy is to *improve the quality of communication* among family members. Specific communication skills are taught according to the procedures of social skills training (as outlined in the next section). Communication skills emphasize the importance of clarity, specificity, and brevity, especially in stating requests and feelings. Expression of positive feelings, expression of negative feelings, and compromise and negotiation are frequently taught skills. Family members are assigned to practice skills outside of scheduled sessions as homework. Satisfactory completion of homework and active role-playing in the session are used as indicators to judge the progress of family members in mastering new skills.

When family members have demonstrated improvement in their communication skills, the next step is to train the family to *solve problems together.* A sequence of problem-solving skills is taught:

1. Define the problem to patient's and family's satisfaction.
2. Brainstorm possible solutions.
3. Evaluate the advantages and disadvantages of each solution.
4. Select the best solution or combination of solutions.
5. Plan on how to implement the solution.
6. After implementation, review progress made toward problem resolution, and conduct additional problem solving as necessary.

The purpose of problem-solving training is to teach the skills families need to solve problems, not to solve specific problems. Initially, the clinician helps family members to learn the problem-solving model by working on small, easily managed difficulties. Later, over time, as family members' problem-solving skills develop, the family proceeds to issues that are more complex and challenging. A critical goal of the behavioral family therapy model is to promote the ability of families to solve problems on their own with minimal help from professionals.

In the final component of behavioral family therapy, the clinician helps family members *develop additional strategies for dealing with problems that remain unresolved.* For example, contingency management, relaxation training, and supplementary skills training may be taught to help family members reduce arousal levels and susceptibility to aggressive episodes.

Controlled research provides strong support for the efficacy of behavioral family therapy for patients with schizophrenia (Falloon et al. 1985; Randolph et al. 1994; Tarrier et al. 1989), and preliminary findings with bipolar disorder patients have also been promising (Miklowitz and Goldstein 1990). The effects of behavioral family therapy on relapse and rehospitalization have been marked. Since violence often occurs during the height of a psychotic episode, the effects of behavioral family therapy on reducing relapses may also reduce violent behavior.

Social Skills Deficits

Clinical strategies that address skills deficits assume that aggressive behavior is a consequence of inadequate interpersonal skills for managing conflict situations and expressing angry feelings (Bornstein et al. 1985). For example, a patient who is angered by another person but who lacks the interpersonal skills for appropriately conveying that anger may resort to violence when the frustration becomes too great to bear. Teaching more effective and less destructive social skills may decrease violent episodes of behavior.

Interpersonal skills can be taught using the techniques of social skills training (Liberman et al. 1989). Social skills training is a structured approach to teaching skills to psychiatric patients that is grounded in social-learning theory (Bandura 1969). The training is conducted either individually or in groups following a standardized curriculum. Social-learning theory in groups is conducted in the following sequence:

1. Establish a rationale for learning the skill.
2. Break the skill into component steps.
3. Model the skill in a role-play for participating patients.
4. Review with the patients what they observed in the role-play.
5. Engage one patient in a role-play to practice the skill.
6. Provide positive feedback about components of the skill that were performed well.
7. Provide corrective feedback regarding how patients could do the skill better.

8. Engage patients in another role-play of the same situation, provide additional feedback, and conduct more role-plays as necessary.
9. Assign homework to practice the skill.

A variety of different social skills can be taught to psychiatric patients to reduce aggressive behavior (Douglas and Mueser 1990). Some of the most commonly taught skills include expressing negative feelings, compromise and negotiation, problem solving, and assertiveness skills. For example, Charlie learns assertiveness by directly stating how a person's actions intrude upon his personal space. This may require expressing negative feelings about the person's actions. Charlie also learns compromise and problem-solving skills when he must find some middle ground with the other person to avoid a larger battle. Social skills training programs vary in their length, usually ranging from several months to more than a year in duration, depending on severity of the psychiatric disorder and the aggressive behavior.

Research clearly supports the efficacy of social skills training for patients with severe mental illness. There is accumulating evidence across numerous controlled studies that social skills training has beneficial effects on the course of psychiatric disorders (Lehman and Steinwachs 1994; Mueser et al. 1995). The effects of social skills training appear to be most prominent on improving social functioning, although some reports also indicate a reduced vulnerability to relapse.

Cognitive Skills

While the purpose of traditional social skills training is primarily changing behavior, the purpose of newer skills training programs is to address cognitive factors that may have an impact on behavior. Cognitive-behavioral interventions for anger problems in psychiatric patients have applied Novaco's cognitive model of anger (Novaco 1975). According to this model, anger and aggression are mediated by an individual's perception of threat from others and his or her ability to formulate strategies for managing conflict in a nonaggressive manner. Teaching individuals how to cope more effectively with their anger has the following components:

1. Training individuals to recognize their unique early signs of anger so they are more aware of when they need to use anger management skills
2. Teaching patients to recognize potentially provocative situations and to identify nonaggressive responses, such as problem solving

3. Providing a repertoire of behavioral skills for managing conflict, such as walking away

For example, Harry realized he paces and speaks loudly when he is angry. Harry knows he paces and speaks loudly at work when he is tired at the end of the day and he feels his partner, Joe, is not doing his fair share. Rather than blow up at Joe, Harry has learned to take a short break before the last half hour of work. This cooling off period alone in the lunchroom has helped him avoid several outbursts.

Incentives to Use Skills

Some psychiatric patients need to be motivated to change and become less aggressive. Therefore, if skills training programs are to be effective, incentives must be provided for the use of these skills, and response costs must be attached to aggressive behavior.

Social reinforcement of newly acquired skills in the natural environment, at the patients' residence or on the wards, is an incentive that is critical to maintaining new skills. Skills instructors can ensure social reinforcement by periodically meeting with care providers to review skills taught to reduce aggression. For example, therapists might meet with a mother and father to coach them to praise their son or daughter whenever he or she practices anger-reduction skills. This strategy tends to increase the likelihood that care providers will encourage use of social skills for managing conflict situations. Care providers may also learn to prompt patients to choose the most appropriate targeted skill for a particular situation.

Motivation can also be provided by posting the steps of the critical skills in prominent locations where patients can see them. Psychiatric patients often have cognitive deficits, including poor memory, that may interfere with their ability to remember requisite skills. By being provided reminders, patients may be able to use skills that they might otherwise have forgotten.

Intervention Strategies for Disruptive and Aggressive Behavior

Acceleration of Aggression

Behavioral strategies can help patients learn nonviolent responses to frustration and interpersonal conflict, but assaultive incidents may still occur on inpatient units and must be addressed. Behavior therapists have created a hierarchy of intervention strategies designed to stop assaults, remove secondary gains, and, in some instances, provide learning opportunities to acquire alternative responses (American Psychiatric Association 1984; Corrigan et al. 1993). These strategies are summarized in hierarchical order in Table 4–2. Responses in the hierarchy are ranked from least intrusive (i.e., those with the least risk of physical injury or humiliation) to most intrusive (i.e., those posing greater risks). Staff on inpatient units must establish criteria for choosing among various strategies. The choice of strategy is facilitated by a review of the patient's problems and reactions to past interventions. Whenever possible, clinicians should select the least restrictive and risky intervention.

Table 4–2. Behavioral techniques that decelerate aggressive behavior

Strategy	Indication
Social extinction	Effective before violence occurs with patients who respond to social reinforcers
Contingent observation	Effective before violence occurs with patients who respond to social reinforcers
Self-controlled time-out	Effective with violent patients immediately after incidents
Overcorrection	Effective with relatively docile patients
Contingent restraint	Effective with violent patients who do not comply with self-controlled time-out and are resistant to guided practice

Note. Techniques are listed hierarchically, with the more intrusive interventions listed toward the bottom of the table.

Decelerative techniques are punitive in nature and therefore are likely to reduce the frequency of targeted behaviors quickly. These decrements, however, will only be maintained if reinforcing strategies—those that teach the patients coping skills that they might adopt instead of aggression—are paired with the decelerative strategy.

Social Extinction

Many patients like to talk with staff members. Hence, withdrawal of staff attention when these patients exhibit aggressive behaviors may decrease the rate of future aggression, especially if evidence suggests that the violent outburst is maintained by attention from peers or staff.

Extinction is most commonly used with mildly aggressive or disruptive behaviors that do not require immediate staff response (e.g., threatening gestures or loud vocalizations).

Staff explicitly define the target behavior and the amount of time staff will ignore the patient in an effort to extinguish the behavior. For example, staff on Unit 24 decided to ignore Sam every time he had a tantrum because he only got one cup of coffee at afternoon snack time. They would continue ignoring him until he stopped the tantrum for 5 minutes. Effective extinction requires all staff to ignore the designated patient during the intervention. Hence, staff should not discuss the inappropriate behavior with the patient and should avoid eye contact. Staff who were not present when the inappropriate behavior was exhibited should be notified that an extinction schedule has been implemented so that they interact with the patient as other clinicians do.

B. F. Skinner (1953) found that immediately after a target behavior was extinguished, the behavior increased in frequency before diminishing. Applying this finding clinically, one would expect assaultive behaviors that are being extinguished by staff to initially become more severe. For example, Unit 24 staff noticed that Sam's tantrums actually got worse when the staff first started to ignore him. Staff need to be taught this point so that they do not prematurely relinquish the intervention strategy. If used consistently, extinction may be an effective means to diminish the rate of inappropriate behaviors (Liberman et al. 1974).

Contingent Observation

Although social extinction may decrease tantrums and threats, it does not provide an opportunity to learn alternative responses to frustration and conflict. Clinicians using contingent observation instruct patients who are acting out to sit quietly for a predefined time on the perimeter of a group (Porterfield et al. 1976). While sitting alone, patients are instructed to watch peers and staff carefully and to observe alternative responses they might use to avoid future angry responses in the situation. For example, Sam was instructed to sit along the wall of the snack room and watch how other patients deal with only getting one cup of coffee. Staff verbally reinforce the patient when he or she is quietly watching others. Moreover, staff query the patient about what he or she may have observed from others: "Sam, you may have noticed that Harry wanted a second cup of coffee. How did he handle it?" The observation period continues until the patient remains calm for 2 minutes, at which time he or she may return to the group.

Self-Controlled Time-Out

Time-out from reinforcement is an operant technique in which socially inappropriate and/or aggressive behaviors are decreased by separating the patient from overstimulating (and perhaps reinforcing) situations. For example, Mary frequently became loud and angry at clubhouse parties when the room became crowded and the radio loud. She calmed down noticeably when she stepped into her case manager's office for a few minutes' break.

Time-out is most effective for patients who experience loss of social contact as punitive. Self-controlled time-out is not like seclusion, however, because it evokes less resistance (Glynn et al. 1989). Patients have much more control over the time-out process. In this way, time-out offers a less restrictive alternative to seclusion and restraints, engenders less humiliation, and poses less risk of injury.

To implement the procedure, staff prompt aggressive patients to enter time-out. Staff on an inpatient unit may tape off one corner of a quiet, low-traffic room where patients are instructed to "time-out." Patients are told to remain in the quiet area until they have been nonaggressive for 2 minutes. Sometimes continued aggression in the time-out area may result in a lengthy intervention. However, time-out periods that are excessive (over an hour) become overly punitive and diminish the purpose of the intervention. Patients who do not comply with time-out instructions after 1 minute are told to enter the seclusion room. Hence, seclusion is used as a punisher for patients who do not comply with the time-out promptly.

Overcorrection

Overcorrection combines time-out and an effort requirement to reduce the rate of offensive behaviors by forcefully replacing these behaviors with more prosocial alternatives (Foxx and Azrin 1972; Ollendick and Matson 1978). The effort requirement compels patients to restore the disturbed situation to a vastly improved condition. For example, a patient who hit someone might be required to apologize to the victim, the other patients on the ward, and the staff.

Frequently, gentle force may be necessary to guide the patient toward beginning the task. A patient who throws soda in the dayroom may be physically guided to pick up a sponge and wash the wall thoroughly. Only the minimum force necessary to implement the overcorrection procedure should be used. Although manual guidance may at first be necessary to establish instructional control, the procedure is contraindicated for patients who repeatedly refuse to participate after the initial guidance period. Extreme caution with this approach is warranted; any coercive program applied to recalcitrant patients may escalate into incidents of staff injury or patient abuse.

Contingent Restraint

Contingent restraint is operationally similar to conventional restraining methods (see Chapter 6, this volume), with a few differences. It demands immediate and consistent administration of restraint after each episode of severe violence. Moreover, staff do not interact verbally with patients during restraints so as not to reinforce inadvertently the maladaptive behavior.

Conclusion

Behavior therapy provides a broad range of interventions that help patients avoid and contain aggression. Three groups of strategies were reviewed in this chapter: strategies that provide structure for the milieu, help patients replace aggressive behaviors with more prosocial responses, and help them to decelerate their aggression. Incentive strategies like the token economy provide significant structure to the therapeutic milieu. The prescription of explicit interpersonal rules (e.g., "If you go to group, then you receive 10 tokens; you may use these tokens to purchase a snack at 3:00") decreases possible frustrations among patients as well as between patients and staff. Clearly defined rules help the cognitively disabled individual to better understand the social environment, thereby avoiding problems that arise when patients misunderstand another's intentions.

Different behavioral strategies also help decelerate aggressive behaviors. These strategies were hierarchically arranged in this chapter so that clinicians might begin with the least intrusive of interventions; strategies like these pose the least risk for staff and aggressive patient alike. Staff may move to more intrusive interventions when needed. Decelerative techniques frequently obviate the need for emergency medication and restraints.

Perhaps the most useful set of behavioral strategies are those that help the patient replace aggressive behaviors with more adaptive interventions. Basic social skills training helps individuals meet interpersonal needs in a prosocial manner. Through assertion training and problem solving, patients are taught how to get their needs met in a mutually respectful manner.

Behavioral strategies are notable for their specificity and potency.

Much like drug treatments, specific behavioral treatments are indicated for specific aggressive actions. They often have a quick and noticeable impact. Therefore, the treatment team needs to master a broad range of behavioral treatments for the breadth of aggressive behaviors that disrupt inpatient units.

References

American Psychiatric Association: Behavior analysis and therapy and restrictive procedures, in Seclusion and Restraint: The Psychiatric Uses (Task Force Report 22). Washington, DC, American Psychiatric Association, 1984

Asarnow RF, Asamen J, Granholm E, et al: Cognitive/neuropsychological studies of children with a schizophrenic disorder. Schizophr Bull 20:647–669, 1994

Bandura A: Principles of Behavior Modification. New York, Holt, Rinehart, and Winston, 1969

Birchwood M, Smith J, MacMillan F, et al: Predicting relapse in schizophrenia: the development and implementation of an early signs monitoring system using patients and families as observers. A preliminary investigation. Psychol Med 19:649–656, 1989

Bornstein PH, Weisser CE, Balleweg BJ: Anger and violent behavior, in Handbook of Clinical Behavior Therapy With Adults. Edited by Hersen M, Bellack AS. New York, Plenum, 1985, pp 603–629

Bushman BJ, Cooper HM: Effects of alcohol on human aggression: an integrative research review. Psychol Bull 107:341–354, 1990

Cascardi M, Mueser KT, DeGiralomo J, et al: Physical aggression against psychiatric inpatients by family members and partners. Psychiatr Serv 47:531–533, 1996

Corrigan PW: Use of a token economy with seriously mentally ill patients: criticisms and misconceptions. Psychiatr Serv 46:1258–1263, 1995

Corrigan PW, Yudofsky SC, Silver JM: Pharmacological and behavioral treatments for aggressive psychiatric inpatients. Hospital and Community Psychiatry 44:125–133, 1993

Douglas MS, Mueser KT: Teaching conflict resolution skills to the chronically mentally ill: social skills training groups for briefly hospitalized patients. Behav Modif 14:519–547, 1990

Estroff SE, Zimmer C, Lachicotte WS, et al: The influence of social networks and social support on violence by persons with serious mental illness. Hospital and Community Psychiatry 45:669–684, 1994

Falloon IRH, Boyd JL, McGill CW, et al: Family management in the prevention of morbidity of schizophrenia: clinical outcome of a two-year longitudinal study. Arch Gen Psychiatry 42:887–896, 1985

Foxx RM, Azrin NH: Restitution: a method of eliminating aggressive-disruptive behavior of retarded and brain damaged patients. Behav Res Ther 10:15–27, 1972

Glynn SM, Bowen LL, Marshall BD, et al: Compliance with less restrictive aggression-control procedures. Hospital and Community Psychiatry 40:82–84, 1989

Lehman AF, Steinwachs DM: Literature Review: Treatment Approaches for Schizophrenia. Baltimore, MD, Schizophrenia Patient Outcomes Research Team (PORT), University of Maryland, 1994

Liberman RP, Wallace CJ, Teigen J, et al: Interventions with psychotic behaviors, in Innovative Treatment Methods in Psychopathology. Edited by Calhoun KS, Adams HE, Mitchell KM. New York, Wiley, 1974, pp 110–149

Liberman RP, DeRisi WJ, Mueser KT: Social Skills Training for Psychiatric Patients. New York, Pergamon, 1989

Lukoff D, Ventura J, Nuechterlein KH, et al: Integrating symptom assessment into psychiatric rehabilitation, in Handbook of Psychiatric Rehabilitation. Edited by Liberman RP. New York, Macmillan, 1992, pp 56–77

Miklowitz DJ, Goldstein MJ: Behavioral family treatment for patients with bipolar affective disorder. Behav Modif 14:457–489, 1990

Mueser KT, Glynn SM: Behavioral Family Therapy for Psychiatric Disorders. Needham Heights, MA, Allyn & Bacon, 1995

Mueser KT, Wallace CJ, Liberman RP: New developments in social skills training. Behaviour Change 12:31–40, 1995

Novaco RW: Anger Control: The Development and Evaluation of an Experimental Treatment. Lexington, MA, Lexington Books, 1975

Nuechterlein KH, Dawson ME, Gitlin M, et al: Developmental processes in schizophrenic disorders: longitudinal studies of vulnerability and stress. Schizophr Bull 18:387–425, 1992

Ollendick TH, Matson JL: Overcorrection: an overview. Behavior Therapy 9:830–842, 1978

Paul GL, Lentz RJ: Psychosocial Treatment of Chronic Mental Patients: Milieu Versus Social-Learning Programs. Cambridge, MA, Harvard University Press, 1977

Porterfield JK, Herbert-Jackson E, Risley TR: Contingent observation: an effective and acceptable procedure for reducing disruptive behavior of young children in a group setting. J Appl Behav Anal 9:55–64, 1976

Randolph ET, Eth S, Glynn S, et al: Behavioral family management in schizophrenia: outcome from a clinic-based intervention. Br J Psychiatry 164:501–506, 1994

Skinner BF: Science and Human Behavior. New York, Free Press, 1953

Spaulding WD, Reed D, Poland J, et al: Cognitive deficits in psychotic disorders, in Cognitive Rehabilitation for Neuropsychiatric Disorders. Edited by Corrigan PW, Yudofsky SC. Washington, DC, American Psychiatric Press, 1996, pp 129–166

Straznickas KA, McNiel DE, Binder RL: Violence toward family caregivers by mentally ill relatives. Hospital and Community Psychiatry 44:385–387, 1993

Tardiff K: Characteristics of assaultive patients in private hospitals. Am J Psychiatry 141:1232–1235, 1984

Tarrier N, Barrowclough C, Vaughn C, et al: Community management of schizophrenia: a two-year follow-up of a behavioral intervention with families. Br J Psychiatry 154:625–628, 1989

Torrey EF, Taylor EH, Bracha HS, et al: Parental origin of schizophrenia in a subgroup of discordant monozygotic twins. Schizophr Bull 20:423–432, 1994

CHAPTER 5

A Social-Learning Approach to Reducing Aggressive Behavior Among Chronically Hospitalized Psychiatric Patients

Anthony A. Menditto, Ph.D.
Niels C. Beck, Ph.D.
Paul Stuve, Ph.D.

Aggression is a very serious problem within public psychiatric facilities, but its treatment and management have long been a controversial issues (Appelbaum 1983; Fisher 1994). The most common approaches belong to one of three general categories: pharmacotherapy, physical restraints and seclusion, and psychosocial treatments. In this chapter we focus on psychosocial treatments based on learning theory. *Learning theory* is concerned with observable behavior rather than underlying feelings or unconscious motivations. Its most basic principle is that the frequency of behavior is a function of its consequences. When a person's behavior has a positive result for that person, the behavior is more likely to occur again.

In this chapter we illustrate how learning-based treatment techniques can be implemented at a large inpatient facility as we describe a comprehensive treatment program for chronically institutionalized adults at Fulton State Hospital. The program has demonstrated efficacy in increasing desirable and adaptive behaviors and decreasing maladaptive and dangerous behaviors such as assault.

Learning-Based Treatment Techniques

The usefulness of learning-based treatment techniques for individuals with severe and persistent mental disorders has a line of documented empirical support dating back nearly three decades (for reviews, see Fuoco and Tyson 1986; Glynn 1990; Glynn and Mueser 1986; Kazdin 1985; Liberman 1988; Paul and Lentz 1977; Paul and Menditto 1992). This research is rooted in laboratory-based experiments on learning. Early applications of operant reinforcement in inpatient facilities can be seen in published reports of token economies (Atthowe and Krasner 1968; Ayllon and Azrin 1968). In these programs, staff used tokens, such as special cards or chips, to reinforce appropriate patient behaviors. Tokens could then be used to acquire valued goods or privileges. These early programs were particularly successful at enhancing patient self-care skills and socialization as well as at increasing discharge rates. Further-more, numerous reports have documented the effectiveness of learning-based techniques in reducing aggression among institutionalized patients (e.g., Foxx and Azrin 1972; Matson and Stephens 1977; Repp and Deitz 1974; Wong et al. 1985). However, many early inpatient appli-cations of learning-based techniques focused on a limited range of patient problem behaviors, were plagued with problems in staff consis-tency in the execution of techniques, and did not always result in gener-alization of acquired skills into novel situations outside of the hospital. The comprehensive social-learning program, which evolved from this line of research, expanded the range of learning-based procedures to apply to all problematic aspects of patient functioning, developed super-visory structures and processes to enhance staff consistency, and included extensive generalization training.

In a landmark 6-year study, Paul and Lentz (1977) compared the effectiveness of a comprehensive social-learning program, a milieu-therapy program, and traditional hospital treatment for severely regressed and floridly psychotic chronically hospitalized psychiatric patients. The social-learning program included techniques based on learning theory that were systematically applied to all patient problem behaviors throughout a rich schedule of treatment activities. Addition-ally, it included an elaborate token-economy structure and generaliza-tion training. The milieu-therapy program was as active and compre-hensive as the social-learning program and was based on the most successful applications of the milieu-therapy approach at that time (Cumming and Cumming 1962; Ellsworth 1968; Fairweather 1964; Jones 1968; Kraft 1966; Paul 1969). This program included an active treatment schedule of wardwide and small-group interventions, a therapeutic community structure, with an emphasis on social group pressure for improvement, clear conveyance by staff of expectations for appropriate behavior, and a focus on socialization experiences. The same group of staff implemented both the social-learning program and the milieu-

therapy program to control for potential confounds due to staff characteristics. Staff were rigorously trained in each program. Their functioning
was continuously monitored in order to ensure that they adhered to
program principles and procedures. The traditional hospital program
was primarily custodial in nature, with a heavy reliance on biomedical
treatments.

The results of this project were very clear: the social-learning
program was more effective and cost-efficient than either the milieu-
therapy program or traditional hospital treatment at bringing about
improvements in all areas of both adaptive and maladaptive patient
functioning, including aggressive behavior. Also, more patients were
successfully discharged from the social-learning program than from
either of the other two approaches during the study period. Although
not explicitly designed as an "aggression management program," the
social-learning program included interventions that were effective in
dealing with patients who engaged in frequent violent acts, a primary
clinical problem among a significant portion of the population investigated.

On the basis of the Paul and Lentz (1977) results, Fulton State
Hospital adopted the social-learning approach as its "treatment of
choice" for chronically institutionalized patients in both the Forensic and
General Adult Psychiatric Services of the hospital. The remainder of this
chapter is devoted to describing the program, how it addresses the difficult problem of aggressive behavior among severely disabled inpatients,
and how it has succeeded.

Overview of a
Social-Learning Program

The social-learning approach holds that patients either have never
learned or have forgotten adaptive interpersonal, instrumental-role, and
self-care skills. Its goals are learning everyday skills such as grooming
and conversation, increasing performance at work and in home management, decreasing or stopping bizarre and dangerous behavior, and
enhancing community living and problem-solving skills. To attain these
goals, patients participate in a structured program of self-care training,
classes, groups, recreational and social activities, and vocational
training.

Patient performance is continually monitored and fostered by differential reinforcement. Throughout the day, staff observe and interact with
patients to influence their behavior. They reinforce desirable, but not

undesirable, behaviors, providing prompts (e.g., "If you get out of bed on time, you will get a token") and immediate execution of specified consequences. Appropriate behavior is reinforced with tokens, shaping chips, praise, and warm social interaction. Tokens are small, square slips of paper that are given to patients when they meet individualized performance targets. The tokens can be exchanged for a wide variety of goods and privileges.

Shaping chips look just like tokens, but they cannot be exchanged for anything. Rather, they are used as concrete reinforcers for behaviors that will lead to token reinforcement. In other words, shaping chips are used to bridge the gap between discrete appropriate behaviors and eventually earning a token. Thus, when patients earn a shaping chip (at which time they also receive praise and encouragement), they know that if they continue appropriate performance they will earn a token.

The system by which patients earn and spend tokens is referred to as a *token economy*. Token economies have a long documented history of effectiveness with hospitalized psychiatric patients (Ayllon and Azrin 1968; Glynn 1990; Kazdin 1985). The social-learning program includes an elaborate token economy that governs access to a wide range of goods, privileges, and services. Patients have numerous opportunities throughout the day both to earn and to spend tokens (Table 5–1). In many ways the token economy resembles a monetary economy in the community. While creating an incentive for patients to participate in their treatment, it also affords them opportunities to make choices and take more responsibility for their lives, as they will be required to do in the community.

In conjunction with the token economy, the social-learning program has four step levels. At step 1, patients are generally still engaging in high rates of bizarre and/or aggressive behavior. The major focus at this step is on meeting minimal behavioral expectations and decreasing aggression. When patients are at step 2, the treatment emphasis begins to shift toward higher-level social and vocational skills. At steps 3 and 4, there is an even stronger emphasis on the vocational training and skills and supports necessary for transitioning into the community.

As patients progress through the step levels they can earn more tokens, and so gain access to more goods and privileges. However, token payment for vocational training activities at steps 2 and 3 is delayed and given as a weekly paycheck. Payment is done in this way to begin the process of delaying gratification and enhancing generalization and maintenance of appropriate behavior. At step 4, tokens are eliminated from the program altogether and patients receive a weekly credit card

Table 5–1. Examples of ways tokens are earned and spent in a social-learning program

Ways to earn tokens	Ways to spend tokens	
Get up on time	**One token**	**Four tokens**
Attend groups, classes, activities	Penny candy	Snack cake
Participate in community meeting	Audiocassette tape rental	Wallet
Complete housekeeping chores	Audio tape player rental	Watchband
Participate in vocational training	Private TV/stereo	Playing cards
Meet individual performance targets for:	Room (30 minutes)	**Five tokens**
Appearance checks (3 times/day)	**Two tokens**	Batteries
Bed and area checks	Instant coffee	Popcorn
Bathing checks	Small box of candy	Headphones
Meal behavior (3 times/day)	Smoking privilege	Chips/pretzels
Participation in groups, classes, and activities	Greeting card	Cheeseburger
(5–7/day)	Soup	Diet fruit snacks
Participation in informal interaction periods	Leisure event pass	Poster
(2–4/day)	**Three tokens**	**Six tokens**
	Extra stamps	Candy bar
	Ice cream	Aftershave
	Burrito	**Twelve tokens**
	Hot dog	Watch
	Movie night (includes soda and snack)	

that entitles them to a great many goods and privileges. As patients transition into the community, the credit card is eliminated and patients acquire goods with their own personal funds. If a patient engages in an aggressive act at any step level, he or she is automatically demoted to step 1.

Consistency and predictability across time and staff members are keys to the treatment program. For patients, behavioral expectations and consequences must always be clear. Rules are stated in simple, unambiguous language and posted in common areas. Staff continually monitor and record patient behavior, using descriptive language such as "Mr. Jones was frequently changing positions in his seat. He was also seen repeatedly pulling his hair and picking at small lesions on his arm" rather than inferential language such as "Mr. Jones was upset and anxious." They record actual patient behaviors, desired behaviors, tokens and shaping chips earned, and tokens spent.

In the social-learning program, staff provide guidance and encouragement rather than taking on a critical or punitive role. Most of their interactions with patients are positive because they take pains to provide opportunities for adaptive behaviors and to reinforce them. The delivery of shaping chips and tokens is always paired with social praise and encouragement. Behavior that is not desirable but not against the rules is generally ignored in order to facilitate its extinction. Behavior that is against the rules, including, of course, dangerous behavior, is subject to response costs. These consist of token fines and may include brief periods of time-out from reinforcement.

Differential Reinforcement

To create an environment that can facilitate skill development on an inpatient ward, staff differentially reinforce behaviors that are adaptive and incompatible with aggression and ignore or apply negative consequences to maladaptive behaviors (Ball 1993; Paul and Lentz 1977; Wong et al. 1985). This may seem simple, but it can be very difficult to accomplish sufficient procedural consistency—both with the same staff member at different times and across different staff members—for these techniques to be effective. Staff must also provide timely reinforcement (usually immediately following appropriate behavior) with a high degree of behavioral specificity to avoid inadvertently reinforcing maladaptive behavior. To meet these ends, staff are provided extensive training and considerable monitoring and supervision in procedures based on operant and associative learning principles. Differential reinforcement constitutes a network of structured interactions between staff and patients that supports and expands upon skills training classes and groups.

Throughout the day patients receive frequent positive reinforcement with shaping chips, tokens, and verbal praise when they demonstrate adaptive behaviors. Examples of desirable behaviors include appropriately conversing with others, playing cooperative games, grooming, participating in structured activities, and resolving conflict without aggression. On the other hand, they are usually ignored when they engage in bizarre or unusual behaviors that are not against the rules. Staff may remind a patient that bizarre behavior will result in losing a chance to earn a token. If the behavior ceases and the patient engages in appropriate behavior, he or she will be praised and encouraged. If the behavior continues, there will be no further prompts; it will be completely ignored. When patients exhibit behaviors that violate rules or pose a danger to others, there are required response costs.

The use of differential reinforcement is facilitated by prompts: direct statements to patients that clarify behavioral expectations and consequences. Positive prompts specify behaviors that will result in positive consequences—for example, "Jim, you've done a very good job combing your hair. Now, if you shave, you will be able to earn a token." Negative prompts point out behaviors that will result in negative consequences if they continue. An example is, "Charlie you are beginning to raise your voice and yell at Mike. If you keep yelling like that, you will have to go to time-out and be fined 10 tokens." Negative prompts should always be paired with positive prompts, as follows: "Now Charlie, if you will calm down and lower your voice, we'll be able to discuss your concerns and hopefully work this thing out between you and Mike. Then the two of you can stay friends, and you will be able to go to your next class, which starts in a few minutes, and earn a token." By consistently delivering prompts and following through with the consequences they promise, staff are able to provide guidance without becoming authoritarian. Patients can then choose their own behavior and its consequences, which is critical for learning.

Shaping

Patients in the social-learning program have individualized behavioral targets or goals that change as their behavior improves. Targets become more difficult to achieve so that they continue to provide a challenge for continued improvement but remain within the individual patient's capability. For example, at the start of a basic conversation skills class, a patient may receive a shaping chip each time he or she makes a statement that is related to the topic at hand and reality based, and a token when this is done three times. Once the patient has mastered this level of participation, he or she must make two appropriate statements to earn a shaping chip and six statements in each class to earn a token. Targets are shifted until the patient is able to sustain appropriate participation throughout the class. In the same class, another, higher-functioning patient may have more advanced behavioral goals. The second patient may be required to actively participate in and attend to the class discussion for 10 minutes to earn a shaping chip and to do so throughout the class to earn a token. As patients progress through the program, the use of tokens is systematically faded and eventually eliminated altogether to provide for generalization and maintenance of acquired skills.

Response-Cost Procedures

Inappropriate or dangerous behaviors are addressed with a three-tiered infraction system of token fines and time-out from reinforcement. Relatively minor rule violations, such as using goods or services without paying tokens, incur a 5-token fine. More serious behaviors—those that infringe on the rights of others, such as public masturbation, cursing at others, and stealing—result in a 10-token fine and a 15-minute period of time-out from reinforcement. Acts of violence or threats of violence are considered "intolerable behaviors." They are followed by a 25-token fine and time-out or seclusion depending on the patient's level of dangerousness. In all cases, patients cannot purchase any goods or privileges until token fines are paid.

This clearly delineated infraction system can reduce the frequency of aggressive behavior in several ways. First, both behaviors and consequences are clearly specified so that patients can comprehend their predictable relationships. The development of such an understanding is essential to learning. Second, by consistently executing the procedures for less serious behaviors, many escalations into actual aggression are avoided. Third, because patients obtain nearly all goods and privileges through a carefully monitored token economy, response-cost procedures are more meaningful to patients and thereby more effective. This is especially true for intolerable behaviors that, because of their seriousness, have a severe response cost. (The 25-token fine represents most patients' average daily earning potential.) Finally, because of the extremely high rates of ongoing reinforcement in the social-learning program, time-out procedures truly mean "time-out from reinforcement." The rate of verbal reinforcement across staff members in the program averages more than 40 instances per hour. Additionally, patients receive shaping chips and tokens throughout the day, and they have numerous opportunities to purchase goods and privileges with tokens. When removed from such a rewarding environment and placed in time-out, a patient is more likely to appreciate and respond to loss of reinforcement.

Skills Training

The social-learning program is not merely an elaborate contingency management system. Rather, the program offers a wide range of ongoing skills training classes and groups (Table 5–2) designed to empower patients with adaptive interpersonal skills that can substitute for aggressive and otherwise maladaptive behaviors.

Table 5–2.   Groups and classes in a social-learning program

Self-care training
Special education classes
Basic conversation skills training
Social skills training
Problem-solving skills group (didactic and experiential)
Basic and advanced life skills training
Leisure and recreational activities
Anger management training
Basic job skills training
Vocational training
Community reintegration training
Prerelease group

Considerable research has documented the effectiveness of such approaches for increasing prosocial behavior and decreasing maladaptive and aggressive behavior in individuals with severe and persistent mental illness (for reviews, see Corrigan et al. 1992; Corrigan and Mueser, Chapter 4, this volume). Skills training is offered through both didactic and experiential groups that are conducted one to three times a week. Patients may be enrolled in these groups for a period of months to years, depending on their individual needs.

In the didactic groups, instructors/therapists attempt to teach patients a broad range of readily applicable interpersonal skills. Topics range from rudimentary conversation skills to stating needs effectively to assertion training and anger management. The groups provide patients with the basic skills they need to interact effectively in social situations without resorting to threats and violence. Skills are taught by breaking them down into manageable behavioral components. For example, the skill of expressing anger toward others without becoming abusive or violent might be broken down into the following components: identify the experience of anger (internal psychophysiological cues), make eye contact and maintain appropriate distance from person causing anger, modulate tone of voice, and state clearly what the person's actions are that are causing the anger (e.g., "It makes me angry when you do . . ."). When working with severely disabled patients who tend to act out impulsively when angry, this sequence could easily take several months to cover in a group that meets three times a week.

Typically, an instructor will begin teaching each component by demonstrating or modeling the appropriate behavior. Patients will then be asked to practice and role-play the same behavior. While patients are practicing and role-playing, instructors provide ongoing instruction, encouragement, praise, and, if necessary, shaping techniques. For example, a patient who has difficulty making eye contact may be praised and receive a shaping chip each time he or she is able to make eye contact for even a few seconds. Because most patients in the social-learning program have severe cognitive impairments, the content of groups is repeated numerous times in order to enhance learning. Homework assignments are included so that patients can practice skills with peers and staff on the ward and during other activities.

In the experiential groups, many of the same methods are applied to real-life problems that patients are having on the ward or at job-training sites. Very often the problems tackled in these groups are interpersonal conflicts and day-to-day frustrations. Patients learn methods to resolve conflicts nonviolently and self-control strategies to substitute for impulsive behavior in the face of frustrating circumstances. The format emphasizes group discussion and brainstorming techniques to assist patients in dealing more effectively with problematic impulses and circumstances. Patients are helped first to monitor and evaluate their behavior and then to develop behavioral action plans. For example, a patient who has had repeated conflicts with a peer at his vocational training workshop brings this problem to the group, complaining that the other patient is teasing and intimidating him. The therapist facilitates a brainstorming session encouraging members to offer solutions for this problem (e.g., ignore the other patient, request a change in assignment, discuss his concerns with staff at the workshop, confront the other patient). Next, each solution is evaluated by the group as to its potential positive and negative consequences. The best possible solution is selected by the patient, who then, with the assistance of other group members, forms a behavioral action plan for implementing the solution. The patient is expected to report back at a later group as to how well the selected solution worked.

Assessment Systems

Three highly refined direct observational assessment systems guide clinical efforts and provide ongoing evaluation of the effectiveness of the social-learning program and its components. Originally, these systems were developed for the Paul and Lentz (1977) investigation, and they have been studied extensively as part of that and other projects.

The first is the Clinical Frequencies Recording System (CFRS; Redfield 1979), an extensive checklist system in which a variety of target behaviors are monitored: grooming and hygiene skills, mealtime behaviors, housekeeping, laundry, attendance and participation in scheduled treatment activities, interpersonal skills, vocational skills, and all purchases with tokens. Inappropriate behaviors, including all instances of threatening and aggressive behaviors, are also recorded. Clinical staff use the CFRS to record data throughout all patient waking hours according to an event-sampling schedule (i.e., recording is triggered by the occurrence of the event or specified behavior). All data for each day are entered into a computer by nightshift staff while patients are sleeping.

Data obtained from the CFRS are summarized in weekly and monthly printouts that are used for a variety of individual and program-wide decisions. A patient's progression through the program's four step levels is determined by CFRS data. Increasing participation and behavioral competence result in advancement to a higher step level. Additionally, CFRS data are used to monitor the effectiveness of specific interventions within the program for individual patients and groups of patients.

The second of the social-learning program assessment systems is the Time-Sample Behavioral Checklist (TSBC; Paul 1987a), a system of planned discrete observations of individual adults in residential-treatment settings. The TSBC yields detailed level-of-functioning information for use in clinical decision making, program evaluation, and quality improvement. TSBC data are collected by a team of highly trained, independent, noninteractive observers whose only job is the collection of such data. On the basis of 2-second observations, they record the presence or absence of each of 69 specific behavioral codes according to highly standardized and meticulously defined coding rules. The 69 behavioral codes are grouped into seven categories: Location (e.g., bedroom, activity area); Physical Position (e.g., sitting, standing); Awake-Asleep status (e.g., eyes open or closed); Facial Expression (e.g., smiling, grimacing); Social Orientation (e.g., alone, with patients); Concurrent Activities (e.g., talking to others, group activity); and Crazy Behavior (e.g., talking to self, posturing).

Each patient on a particular treatment unit is observed during each waking hour 7 days a week through the use of a stratified hourly time-sampling scheme. This type of sampling consists of observations systematically varied over the beginning, middle, and last 20 minutes of each waking hour throughout the week. A typical week consists of about 90–105 such observations per patient. Weekly TSBC computer summaries yield data on each of the 69 specific behavioral codes and 9 higher-order scores, which include a Total Appropriate Behavior Index and a Total Inappropriate Behavior Index.

The last of the three assessment systems is the Staff-Resident Inter-action Chronograph (SRIC; Paul 1988). This instrument focuses on staff behaviors and those staff-patient interactions that constitute treatment on inpatient units. SRIC data are collected by the same cadre of observers who collect data for the TSBC. They code the target staff member's verbal and nonverbal responses to the behavior of patients over the entire duration of a 10-minute observation period. Multiple 10-minute observations occur for each staff member according to a stratified hourly sampling schedule, which ensures representative coverage of all staff members and activities in proportion to their actual occurrence in the program over a 1-week period.

For each staff-patient interaction, behavior is coded according to extremely detailed operational definitions into one of several categories. Patient behavior is coded into five categories: Appropriate (e.g., playing a game of cards with others, combing hair in preparation for an appearance check); Inappropriate Failure (e.g., sleeping during a skills training class); Inappropriate Crazy (e.g., talking to self, assaulting others); Request (e.g., asking for a towel to take a shower); and Neutral. Staff behaviors are coded into one of 21 different categories, examples of which are Positive Verbals (e.g., "Good job!"); Negative Verbals (e.g., "That's gross!"); Positive and Negative Prompts (e.g., "Bob if you come to class now you can earn a token, but if you just sit there in the hall you won't and you'll miss out on our activity today"); Physical Force (e.g., restraining assaultive patients); Ignore/No Response; and Attend/Record/Observe (e.g, doing paperwork).

Computer-generated summaries of SRIC data reveal the levels of activity and effort of individual staff members as well as the extent to which their interactions adhere to the program's principles and procedures. This allows for evaluation of the effectiveness of staff training procedures as well as assistance in individual supervisory processes.

Reliability and validity of the each of these three instruments have been exceptional. In multisite studies, interobserver reliabilities (intraclass correlations) have ranged from 0.94 to 0.97 for the CFRS (Redfield 1979), and typically exceeded 0.98 for the TSBC (Licht and Paul 1987) and 0.95 for the SRIC (Licht et al. 1988). CFRS and TSBC higher-order scores have demonstrated excellent convergent and discriminant validity with other standardized questionnaires and rating scales of patient functioning (Redfield 1979; Mariotto et al. 1987; Paul 1987b).

With such highly refined assessment procedures, treatment interventions can be tailored toward specific behavior problems (e.g., aggression), with ongoing evaluation of both patient progress and treatment procedures. Using these procedures with the timed introduction of treatment interventions, clinicians and researchers can better understand the nature and amount of a particular intervention required to bring about desired behavior change. In settings without this degree of ongoing assessment, the true source of behavior change is often obscure, and substantial resources may be wasted in pursuing treatment options of questionable or only incidental effectiveness.

Program Evaluation Studies

There have been several reports of some of the results of the social-learning program at Fulton State Hospital. Some described increased cognitive/attentional skills (Menditto et al. 1991), decreases in excessive fluid consumption (Baldwin et al. 1992), and wardwide improvements in overall level of functioning (Menditto et al. 1994). Another documented dramatic reductions in the frequency of aggressive behavior among patients on the original maximum-security social-learning ward at Fulton State Hospital (Beck et al. 1991). Results from this study are presented in Figure 5–1. There was a steady decline in the rate of aggressive behavior among a group of 19 severely disabled, chronically institutionalized forensic patients from baseline through the first 2 years of program implementation. A more detailed analysis of Figure 5–1 reveals that during the 3-month baseline period when treatment consisted of an eclectic program, there were 49 acts of aggression. During the early implementation phase of the social-learning program, which took place during months four through six, there were 43 aggressive acts.

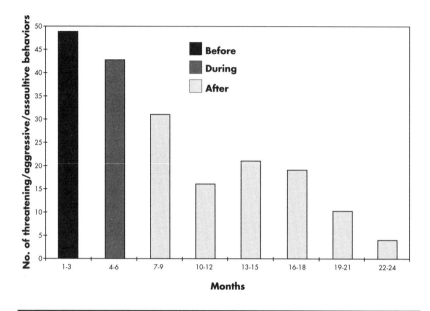

Figure 5–1.   *Frequency of aggressive behaviors among 19 chronically mentally ill forensic patients during 3-month intervals before, during, and after implementation of a social-learning program.*
Source.   *Adapted from Beck NC, Menditto AA, Baldwin LJ, et al.: "Decreasing the Frequency of Aggressive Behavior in Chronically Mentally Ill Forensic Patients."* Hospital and Community Psychiatry 42:750–752, 1991. *Copyright 1991, American Psychiatric Association. Used with permission.*

A Wilcoxon matched-pairs, signed-rank test comparing the frequency of aggressive behavior during the baseline and implementation periods failed to achieve significance at the 0.05 level. Following the program implementation phase, there was a steady decline in the number of threatening, aggressive, or assaultive behaviors (31, 16, 21, 19, 10, and 4, respectively, for each subsequent 3-month period). Additional Wilcoxon tests of the significance of differences between the baseline period and each of six 3-month periods after program implementation all achieved significance at levels that exceeded 0.025. By the last 3-month period in the study, a 92% decrease in aggressive behavior was evident, with only four intolerable acts committed.

Conclusion

The social-learning approach has considerable documented empirical support for use with severely and persistently mentally ill individuals. When used in an inpatient setting, such an approach should include differential reinforcement procedures comprehensively applied to all patient problem behaviors across all waking hours, a tightly controlled token economy, direct skills training components, and direct observational assessment methodology. Programs that include all of these components have reported improvements in all areas of adaptive patient functioning as well as dramatic decreases in maladaptive and inappropriate behaviors, including aggressive acts.

References

Appelbaum PS: Legal considerations in the prevention and treatment of assault, in Assaults Within Psychiatric Facilities. Edited by Lion JR, Reid WH. New York, Grune & Stratton, 1983, pp 173–190

Atthowe JM, Krasner L: Preliminary report on the application of contingent reinforcement procedures (token economy) on a "chronic" psychiatric ward. J Abnorm Psychol 73:37–43, 1968

Ayllon T, Azrin N: The Token Economy: A Motivational System for Therapy and Rehabilitation. New York, Appleton-Century-Crofts, 1968

Baldwin LJ, Menditto AA, Beck NC, et al: Decreasing excessive water drinking behavior in chronically mentally ill forensic patients. Hospital and Community Psychiatry 43:507–509, 1992

Ball GG: Modifying the behavior of the violent patient. Psychiatr Q 64: 359–369, 1993

Beck NC, Menditto AA, Baldwin LJ, et al: Decreasing the frequency of aggressive behavior in chronically mentally ill forensic patients. Hospital and Community Psychiatry 42:750–752, 1991

Corrigan PW, Schade ML, Liberman RP: Social skills training, in Handbook of Psychiatric Rehabilitation. Edited by Liberman RP. Needham Heights, MA, Allyn & Bacon, 1992, pp 95–126

Cumming J, Cumming E: Ego and Milieu. New York, Atherton, 1962

Ellsworth RB: Nonprofessionals in Psychiatric Rehabilitation. New York, Appleton-Century-Crofts, 1968

Fairweather GW (ed): Social Psychology in Treating Mental Illness: An Experimental Approach. New York, Wiley, 1964

Fisher WA: Restraint and seclusion: a review of the literature. Am J Psychiatry 151:1584–1591, 1994

Foxx RM, Azrin NH: Restitution: a method of eliminating aggressive-disruptive behavior of retarded and brain damaged patients. Behav Res Ther 10:15–27, 1972

Fuoco FJ, Tyson WM: Behavior therapy in residential programs for psychiatric clients, in Behavior Analysis and Therapy in Residential Programs. Edited by Fuoco FJ, Christian WP. New York, Van Nostrand Reinhold, 1986, pp 231–259

Glynn SM: Token economy approaches for psychiatric patients: progress and pitfalls over 25 years. Behav Modif 14:383–407, 1990

Glynn SM, Mueser KT: Social learning for chronic mental patients. Schizophr Bull 12:648–668, 1986

Jones M: Beyond the Therapeutic Community: Social Learning and Social Psychiatry. New Haven, CT, Yale University Press, 1968

Kazdin AE: The token economy, in Evaluating Behavior Therapy Outcome. Edited by Turner R, Asher LM. New York, Spring Publishing, 1985, pp 225–253

Kraft AM: The therapeutic community, in American Handbook of Psychiatry (Arieti S, Editor-in-Chief), Vol 3. Edited by Arieti S. New York, Basic Books, 1966, pp 542–551

Liberman RP (ed): Psychiatric Rehabilitation of Chronic Mental Patients. Washington, DC, American Psychiatric Press, 1988

Licht MH, Paul GL: Replicability of TSBC codes and higher-order scores, in Assessment in Residential Treatment Settings, Part 2: Observational Assessment Instrumentation for Service and Research—The Time-Sample Behavioral Checklist. Edited by Paul GL. Champaign, IL, Research Press, 1987, pp 69–94

Licht MH, Paul GL, Mariotto MJ: Replicability of SRIC codes, categories, indexes, and matrix profiles, in Assessment in Residential Treatment Settings, Part 3: Observational Assessment Instrumentation for Service and Research—The Staff-Resident Interaction Chronograph. Edited by Paul GL. Champaign, IL, Research Press, 1988, pp 101–136

Mariotto MJ, Paul GL, Licht MH: Concurrent relationships of TSBC higher-order scores with information from other instruments, in Assessment in Residential Treatment Settings, Part 2: Observational Assessment Instrumentation for Service and Research—The Time-Sample Behavioral Checklist. Edited by Paul GL. Champaign, IL, Research Press, 1987, pp 177–210

Matson JL, Stephens RM: Overcorrection of aggressive behavior in a chronic psychiatric patient. Behav Modif 1:559–564, 1977

Menditto AA, Baldwin LJ, O'Neal LG, et al: Social-learning procedures for increasing attention and teaching basic skills to severely regressed and chronically institutionalized forensic psychiatric patients. J Behav Ther Exp Psychiatry 22:265–269, 1991

Menditto AA, Valdes LA, Beck NC: Implementing a comprehensive social-learning program within the forensic service of Fulton State Hospital, in Behavior Therapy in Psychiatric Hospitals. Edited by Corrigan PW, Liberman RP. New York, Springer, 1994, pp 61–78

Paul GL: Chronic mental patient: current status—future directions. Psychol Bull 71:81–94, 1969

Paul GL (ed): Assessment in Residential Treatment Settings, Part 2: Observational Assessment Instrumentation for Service and Research—The Time-Sample Behavioral Checklist. Champaign, IL, Research Press, 1987a

Paul GL: Discriminations of TSBC higher-order scores among groups differing on clinically relevant characteristics, in Assessment in Residential Treatment Settings, Part 2: Observational Assessment Instrumentation for Service and Research—The Time-Sample Behavioral Checklist. Edited by Paul GL. Champaign, IL, Research Press, 1987b, pp 147–176

Paul GL (ed): Assessment in Residential Treatment Settings, Part 3: Observational Assessment Instrumentation for Service and Research—The Staff-Resident Interaction Chronograph. Champaign, IL, Research Press, 1988

Paul GL, Lentz RJ: Psychosocial Treatment of Chronic Mental Patients: Milieu Versus Social-Learning Programs. Cambridge, MA, Harvard University Press, 1977

Paul GL, Menditto AA: Effectiveness of inpatient treatment programs for mentally-ill adults in public psychiatric facilities. Applied and Preventive Psychology 1:41–63, 1992

Redfield JP: Clinical frequencies recording systems: standardizing staff observations by event recording. Journal of Behavioral Assessment 1:211–219, 1979

Repp AC, Deitz SM: Reducing aggressive and self-injurious behavior of institutionalized retarded children through reinforcement of other behaviors. J Appl Behav Anal 7:313–325, 1974

Wong SE, Slama K, Liberman PR: Behavioral analysis and therapy for aggressive psychiatric and developmentally disabled patients, in Clinical Treatment of the Violent Person. Edited by Roth LH. Rockville, MD, U.S. Department of Health and Human Services, 1985, pp 22–56

SECTION II

Approaches to Understanding Violent Patients

CHAPTER 6

Videotape Recording of Assaults on a Secure Unit of a Large State Psychiatric Hospital

Martha L. Crowner, M.D.

Violence is a great concern to anyone responsible for quality care and safety in psychiatric hospitals. At Manhattan Psychiatric Center, a large New York State facility for the severely mentally ill, assaults on staff and between patients has been a serious problem, but one that has been confronted and alleviated. The facility established a specialized unit for treating violent patients, the Secure Care Unit, and supported a series of research studies to improve the prediction and prevention of violence.

In 1980 the hospital opened the Intensive Psychiatric Service, or IPS, a specialized 14-bed ward with enriched staffing for patients who had been violent at least once while in the hospital. The IPS is designed for quick and intensive treatment followed by return to the home ward. By 1985 it was apparent that a small number of patients had frequent IPS admissions; at that time a second ward with 18 beds was added to the unit, the Intensive Rehabilitation Program, or IRP, for long-term treatment. Later, a third ward with 26 beds was added to complete the configuration of the Secure Care Unit. The unit closed in early 1998.

Over 18 years the unit provided humane and effective treatment for some of the most difficult patients in the hospital. The unit provided clinicians an opportunity to gain extensive experience in treating violent patients. It also afforded an unusual opportunity to undertake formal studies of this population and their behavior. In this chapter I outline the essentials of the organization and function of the Secure Care Unit and present the findings of a series of unique and innovative studies of assaults between inpatients. Finally, drawing on clinical and research experience, I suggest programmatic, administrative, and ward design changes to limit violence on psychiatric wards.

The Secure Care Unit at Manhattan Psychiatric Center

The goal of the Secure Care Unit was to provide treatment and behavioral containment for the most dangerous patients in the hospital. The unit served the entire hospital by removing a select number of patients from large census wards for specialized, intensive care. It has been documented that most inpatient violence is committed by a small percentage of the total population (Convit et al. 1990). Patients were removed from larger wards, where they often disrupted ward milieu and provoked powerful feelings among fellow patients and staff (fear, anger, and helplessness), and offered intensive observation and treatment in a new setting. Most returned to their home wards after brief treatment, but a small minority continued their dangerous behavior and, therefore, remained in the unit. As their functioning gradually improved, they moved on to wards within the unit with fewer restrictions and more responsibilities. The unit offered continuity of care; slow, stepwise progression; and long-term rehabilitation.

Intensive Psychiatric Service

Patients were first admitted to the unit through the IPS, a 14-bed ward for both men and women. The ward functioned in some ways like an admissions unit where patients were assessed, a new treatment plan designed, and its implementation begun; but treatment was targeted at controlling dangerous behavior. Medical staff were attuned to the problems these patients commonly present and adept at managing them. A psychologist and other ward staff implemented psychosocial treatments, including anger management groups and a token-economy system. Therapy aide staff on the unit were specially trained in techniques for calming and restraining violent patients.

The IPS milieu was characterized by closer observation, more restriction, and less stimulation than regular wards. Patients spent most of their waking hours in a large dayroom, where therapy aide staff were in constant attendance. They could not congregate in areas where they could not be observed such as bathrooms and isolated hallways. A large window separated the nurses' station from the dayroom so that nurses and other staff working there could look up and observe patients. Patients did not carry cigarettes or money, which are the objects of many disputes, or belts, shoelaces, matches, metal objects, or glass, which could be used for dangerous purposes. A quiet, gentle, nonconfrontational approach seemed most effective. Staff learned to avoid criticism and to practice tolerance. Patients were prevented from engaging in dangerous and seriously disruptive behavior but otherwise were urged, but not forced, to conform.

The IPS was designed for brief treatment. After patients' symptoms improved and their violent behavior abated, within a few to several weeks, they were usually returned to their home ward, where they were well known, for further stabilization and eventual discharge. A small minority were kept within the unit for longer treatment. Some had had multiple IPS admissions, but without the extra supervision and structure of the Secure Care Unit their behavior deteriorated. Some responded inadequately to medical interventions and continued their assaultiveness, but with decreased frequency.

Step-Down Units

Patients who stayed within the unit moved from the IPS to the IRP, an 18-bed ward also for men and women. The treatment offered was much the same as that on the IPS, but psychosocial interventions, such as the token economy, had a greater role. After patients were better able to function, they moved on to a larger, less structured ward. The third ward was similar to regular wards in that the patients moved about more freely and the census was higher, but ward census was still lower than that in most wards. From this ward patients could be readied for discharge.

Research on Inpatient Violence on the Secure Care Unit After Installation of Video Cameras

In their clinical role, investigators who interviewed violent patients heard many contradictory and unconfirmable accounts: Patients claimed they hit nobody, or that the victim hit first, or that the victim had behaved intolerably and violence was their only recourse. In studies of the incidence of inpatient assault, Brizer et al. (1987) found that, even when staff members witnessed an event, they often had a sketchy impression of what happened. Few could clearly identify precipitants. Some were not even sure who hit whom first. Such inability to provide details about the incident is understandable because physical assaults happen very fast, often when staff members are looking elsewhere.

Video cameras were installed in the dayroom of the IPS to provide information human witnesses could not. These devices enabled investigators to count the number of assaults between patients that occurred in the dayroom, to see what they looked like and what happened just before they occurred, and to compare what patients said happened with what investigators saw happen. In the following subsections, I outline some of the data from a series of studies that followed installation of the video cameras.

How Frequent Is Physical Assault on Psychiatric Wards?

Methods

An early video camera study (Crowner et al. 1994a) compared the number of assaults detected by cameras with the number detected by official incident reports. Video cameras were installed on the IPS in each of the four corners of the dayroom, where patients spent most of their waking hours. They were connected to monitors and videotape recorders that would automatically record when cameras were filming. They were turned on each weekday, except holidays, from 8 A.M. to 12 noon and from 3 to 5 P.M. Investigators reviewed videotapes to detect assaults, here defined as hitting, kicking, slapping, biting, choking, or throwing objects, with definite physical contact between two patients. For comparison, they checked all official reports of assault that occurred in the dayroom during the same time the cameras were running.

Results

During 27 months of videotaping, video cameras were in operation for 3,330 hours. In that time 155 assaults were detected between patients, an average of 1 per 21.48 hours of taping. Incident reports documented only 12 assaults in the dayroom during the same hours. More than 10 times as many assaults were found when video cameras were used as were reported in official incident reports. However, it is important to add that most events that were detected by cameras but not by official reports—125 out of 137 for which we had data—did not result in injuries. A far greater proportion of assaults detected by incident reports, 6 out of 12, resulted in injuries. Video cameras found 6 incidents in which a patient was injured that were not officially documented. We can conclude that on the IPS there were many episodes of hitting, slapping, kicking, and other assaultive behavior that were not documented by incident reports, but that most of this behavior was not injurious.

Discussion

To put this data in perspective, consider another estimate of assault frequency. Lion et al. (1981) also measured incident report sensitivity, but they compared official incident reports with daily ward reports. In their review of reports from 3 months they found almost six times as many physical assaults documented in ward reports as were documented in incident reports (237 vs. 40).

Crowner et al. (1994a), in their videotape study on the IPS reported above, determined the ratio of officially reported to unreported events at Manhattan Psychiatric Center. There was a small number of reported and a large number of unreported assaults when assault was defined strictly as contact such as hitting, punching, kicking, slapping, and so forth. Many of the events detected did not result in injuries, even minor ones. To videotape reviewers, some looked like playful, friendly exchanges of slaps and jabs. Different results are possible if the study had been completed on another ward or at another institution. On the IPS, staff members were virtually always present in the dayroom; if they were not, some of the minor incidents detected by cameras might have progressed to more serious assaults. The rate of reporting varies from institution to institution according to official policy and how that policy is interpreted. Policy at Manhattan Psychiatric Center requires reporting of incidents that result in injury; it is less definite about incidents that do not. It is clear enough, though, from the IPS study and others in the literature, that official incident reports underreport the rate of assault at psychiatric facilities.

What Did the Assaults Look Like, and How Can They Be Described?

The question of what the assaults looked like may seem a strange question, a question with a simple answer, which is that an assault is when somebody gets angry and tries to physically hurt somebody else. But this answer assumes an understanding of patient intent, which can only be known by interview. The video camera investigators did not assume intent; they defined assault in a purely behavioral way, as incidents involving hitting, kicking, slapping, biting, choking, or throwing objects, with unambiguous physical contact. In a later study (Crowner et al. 1995), investigators reviewed the same group of 155 assaults examined in the earlier study (Crowner et al. 1994a) to describe and classify them in a systematic fashion.

Methods

The same group of 155 assaults examined in the earlier study (Crowner et al. 1994a) were classified according to a global judgment of the assailant's intent to hurt. Three classes were created, ranked by degree of assault seriousness. In the least serious class the assailant seemed playful; in the most serious the assailant seemed to try to hurt. In an intermediate group, the assailant did not seem playful or dangerous but seemed to have another motive, perhaps warning the victim. To describe assaults, the investigators also rated three pieces of information from videotapes: force of assailant blows, body area targeted, and reaction of staff in the dayroom. They rated assailant blows as forceful or not forceful, body area targeted as including head and face or body blows only, and staff reactions as none, intervention without separation, separation of combatants, or, rarely, missing (when staff were not present or could not see the event). Assault classification and descriptor ratings were not done independently, but investigators hypothesized that their classification decision was made on the basis of what they saw on videotape (the descriptor information).

For independent, external validation of the meaningfulness of the assault classes, investigators tested the relationship between assault class and presence of injury, detection by incident report, and explanations assailants gave for their behavior.

Results

Of 155 assaults detected, 21 were classified in the least serious group (i.e., assaults that looked like play); 57 were in the intermediate group; and 76 were in the most serious group (i.e., the assailant seemed to try to hurt). One assault could not be classified. Forcefulness of blows, body area targeted, and staff reactions were all related to assault class. Each descriptor variable made an independent significant contribution to assault classification (as determined by multiple logistic regression). Almost all incidents detected by incident report or resulting in injuries were in the most serious class. Assailants' claims that they were playing were significantly associated with the least serious class.

Discussion

Incidents found by incident report, which most hospital administrators are familiar with, are those in the most serious group. The other events have not been described before. All classes of assaultive events involved hitting, kicking, slapping, biting, choking, or throwing objects, but the behavior did not always seem to have the same meaning. The behavior seemed to have different functions, depending on how hard the victim was hit and where; it could be intended to play, to warn, or to hurt. Patients may intend to coerce—to forcefully communicate a wish for the victim to change his or her behavior. The coercion can be accompanied by restraint, so that the victim is warned, or not, so that the victim is hit, slapped, kicked, or punched. The results suggest that IPS patients can show restraint. If they are warning or trying to coerce, they may respond to efforts to teach another way to communicate.

How Do Patients Explain Their Assaults?

The previous study described assailant intent as judged by investigators. How did patient assailants explain their own behavior? This information could help investigators and hospital personnel improve prediction of assaults. Although assault is often described as being "without apparent provocation," it is hard to accept that it comes out of the blue, without warning or provocation and devoid of interpersonal context. A third study was conducted to start to explore several questions: Do certain circumstances or interpersonal interactions predict assault? At times, is there something about the victim's behavior that could be seen as provocative?

Methods

Investigators collected assailants' explanations of their behavior by direct interview (Crowner et al. 1994b). Videotape reviewers provided a research nurse with the name of the assailant, the date and time of the assault, and a brief description of the event. The nurse would approach each patient separately to ask him or her why the assault occurred and record replies verbatim. Many patients refused to offer responses; others offered short, simple replies; still others obliged by discoursing at length and offering multiple reasons for their actions. Replies were later reviewed to discern common themes. All replies were assigned from one to four themes or reasons.

Results

In their explanations of 134 assaults, patients offered 217 reasons, which fell into the following groups (listed in their order of frequency and accompanied by quotations for illustration):

1. *Missing data.* The patient refused to cooperate with the interviewer, or, far less frequently, investigators failed to approach the patient to ask. This category was the one most commonly found, representing 26% of the 217 reasons.
2. *Play (denial of anger or of wanting to hurt).* Twelve percent of the assaultive patients' reasons were categorized as play. "There was nothing serious. I just joke around once in a while." "We were playing. I didn't mean to hit him. I don't feel bad about him."
3. *Insulted.* Twelve percent of the individual explanations were judged to relate to the assaultive patient's feeling insulted. "I couldn't help it. He made me lose face." "She keeps insulting me in front of others. I just did it." "She says bad things about my things. She said my things were not suitable for a man. She always says that I'm crazy."
4. *To get the person to stop doing something.* Nine percent of the reasons were that the assailant was keeping the victim from doing something. "He keeps on bothering me, asking for cigarettes. I just want him to stop. I was only trying to keep him away from me. I did not think of hurting him"
5. *Anger or threats.* Seven percent of the reasons involved expression of anger or a response to perceived threats from the victim. "I was upset. She just ticked me off when she hit me with the ping-pong racket."
6. *Bizarre or psychotic response.* Six percent of the reasons were categorized as relating to a bizarre or psychotic response. "I don't know. I choked her. The voices told me to choke her."
7. *Retaliation.* Six percent of the reasons were classified as representing retaliation. "I defended myself. She hit me. I defended myself. It's just a feeling to fight back. Am I in trouble? Did I do something bad?"
8. *Threatened.* Five percent of reasons expressed the idea that the assaultive patient felt threatened. "He was going to hit my leg, so I hit him." "He said something in Spanish; I didn't understand him."

9. *Denial.* Five percent of the reasons were a simple denial that the assault happened.
10. *Competition.* Four percent of the reasons centered on competition or access to certain items. "He sat on my chair after I stood up to take my medication. I asked him to get up from my chair, but he pretended not to hear me, so I lifted up my chair."
11. *Coercion.* Three percent of the reasons were categorized as getting the victim to do something.
12. *Sexual provocation.* Three percent of the reasons were related to sexual provocation. "He stood up and began talking in Spanish and grabbing his private parts. He wanted me to suck him off. What do you expect me to do? I wanted him to know he couldn't get away with that."

Discussion

It is important to remember that the patients in this study sample did not hold cigarettes or money; this may explain the small number of events that resulted from competition. Also, the events ranged in degree of harmfulness; many were only shoves, pushes, and slaps that did not result in injuries and did not seem intended to do so. Investigators collected explanations for 134 assaults, which were carried out by a relatively small number of patients. Many of the 40 assaultive patients committed only one assault of the 134, whereas others committed several assaults. Moreover, many patients refused comment. These data, then, can only be suggestive.

The results suggest that in many cases the assault did not come out of the blue and was not the result of command hallucinations. Many patient assailants felt provoked by their victims, complaining of some variety of "bothering." It may be that assailants reported an act of the victim that did not occur. Or, it could be that they reported a real event that they perceived in a distorted way because of paranoia. Or, their affective response may have been disproportionate to the provocation because of irritability.

What Happens Just Before an Assault?

With video cameras it is possible to test some of the explanations patients offer for their behavior. Videotape can be reviewed to see if, in fact, the victim's behavior was such that it might be interpreted as a provocation.

Perhaps the victim was threatening, or sitting in the assailant's favorite chair, or insulting.

Victim or assailant behaviors that consistently occur before assaults can be used as predictors. Nursing staff recognize such behaviors; on the basis of experience or intuition, they pick out certain patients to calm or separate from others. Their practice could be based on data as well as intuition and experience. If predictors are to be useful, they must be specific to assault; that is, they must occur significantly more often just before an assault than before randomly selected time periods that do not precede the assault. Useful predictors should also occur early, giving observant ward staff enough time to identify the behaviors and take action.

This line of study may have implications for patient treatment, staff training, and ward design and management. Identifying possible provocations can allow targeted treatment interventions to decrease these behaviors in potential victims. Potential assailants might also learn to respond in nonviolent ways. Psychiatrists may become more aware of the implications of certain symptoms. Psychologists can provide skills training to teach patients nonviolent responses to everyday conflicts with their peers. Managers, designers, and administrators might devise environmental manipulations to minimize interpersonal interactions associated with assault.

Methods

In a fourth video camera study, investigators analyzed the 5 minutes documented on videotape immediately preceding each assault. They reviewed the tape for clearly defined victim and assailant behaviors, or, as they chose to call them, cues. To test for specificity, they chose control segments: 5-minute portions of the tape in which patients were present in the dayroom but no assault occurred. The investigators planned to compare the occurrence of cues in the 5-minute segments just before the assaults with the occurrence of cues in the 5-minute control segments.

Results

The results of this study are still preliminary, but it seems that most of the assaults were preceded by recognizable behaviors from either victim or assailant that were specific to the assault. Four of the behaviors were usually so close in time to the assault that staff could not reasonably be expected to notice and move in time. More useful predictors were threatening gestures (i.e., yelling, fist shaking, pointing, and arguing) and intrusive behaviors (i.e., getting very close, touching, and kissing). These two types of predictive behavior could be targeted to the eventual victim or the assailant, or they could be generalized (i.e., directed to third parties or to no one in particular in the dayroom). When they were not directed to the victim, there was a greater median time between cue and assault.

Discussion

From these preliminary findings it seems that, at least in this population, many patient assaults do not come out of the blue or without apparent provocation or warning. On the contrary, many seem to arise from interpersonal interactions: heated arguments or violations of personal space. It is easy to imply from these interactions that assailants are angry or feeling threatened. This supports some patients' explanations for assaults, which are, that they were bothered, threatened, or retaliating. These findings also suggest that the reasons or precipitants for assault in psychiatric patients may be comparable to those for assault in nonpsychiatric populations. However, the generalizability of the data must be considered in light of our definition of assault. Many of the assaults in this study are non-injurious slaps and pushes, not the incidents that usually cause clinicians great concern.

Recommendations

Secure care experience and video camera studies have many implications for the further study of inpatient violence and for practical ward management. A few practical suggestions can be summarized as follows: watch patients closely, give them space, avoid conflicts between patients, and resolve them early.

One of the key components of care on the IPS is *close patient observation*. Patient census is kept low so that staff can keep track of where all patients are and what they are doing. Staffing levels are sufficient to assign at least one person this job. Staff should be stationed so that they can see patients, and ward space should be designed and managed so that it is easy for staff to do so. On the IPS, patients and many staff members stay in one large room during most of the day—a room visible from the nurses' station through a large window. Camera studies suggest what to look for: yelling, arguing, threatening, and getting too close or touching. Staff can detect cues and intervene quickly in order to prevent an assault or to catch a fight early, before many blows are exchanged, in order to prevent injuries. Staff observing patients should know what to look for and what to do when they see it. They should be specially trained to separate and calm patients, to resolve arguments, and to urge patients to keep their distance.

The IPS has a lower census than regular wards, so patients have more room to move around without bumping into each other. Video camera studies suggest that bumping, jostling, or moving in too close can lead to fights. Hospital staff should remember that patients may interpret events as threatening when most others would not; for example, jostling or crowding may be seen as a homosexual approach. It is important to avoid not only ward overcrowding but also crowding of patients together in small rooms (e.g., for smoking, dining, or other special activities) or regularly requiring them to wait in lines. Medication may be offered by calling each patient individually rather than by requiring them to line up and wait.

Patient explanations suggest that many assaults do not arise spontaneously, but develop from interpersonal conflict. The IPS restriction on free access to cash and cigarettes is designed to prevent conflicts over these much-valued goods, conflicts frequent on other wards. At least for some patients, assaults may be prevented if staff members hold cigarettes and cash and release them on request, when needed. Clinicians should aggressively treat, and perhaps isolate from their peers, those patients who are often victimized or provocative, not just patients who are assaultive. Finally, patients should be encouraged and taught to resolve disputes and grievances nonviolently, through therapeutic community meetings and anger management training.

References

Brizer DA, Convit A, Krakowski M, et al: A rating scale for reporting violence on psychiatric wards. Hospital and Community Psychiatry 38:769–770, 1987

Convit A, Isay D, Otis D, et al: Characteristics of repeatedly assaultive psychiatric inpatients. Hospital and Community Psychiatry 41: 1112–1115, 1990

Crowner ML, Peric G, Stepcic F, et al: A comparison of videocameras and official incident reports in detecting inpatient assaults. Hospital and Community Psychiatry 45:1144–1145, 1994a

Crowner ML, Stepcic F, Peric G, et al: Typology of patient-patient assaults detected by videocameras. Am J Psychiatry 151:1669–1672, 1994b

Crowner M, Peric G, Stepcic F, et al: Psychiatric patients' explanations for assaults. Psychiatr Serv 46:614–615, 1995

Lion JR, Snyder W, Merrill GL: Underreporting of assaults on staff in a state hospital. Hospital and Community Psychiatry 32:497–498, 1981

CHAPTER 7

Violence and Dissociation

A. Jonathan Porteus, M.A.
Zebulon Taintor, M.D.

Our goal in this chapter is to shed some light on the dissociative processes that precede and underlie some violent behavior. The preliminary sections are intended to orient the reader. In the first two sections we define dissociation and provide a prototypical case illustration. The third section is intended to generate an understanding of how the relationship between dissociation and violence emerges by exploring posttraumatic states, psychological and physiological dysregulation, encapsulation and engraving of memory, and some of the neurobiological rudiments of both dissociation and violence. We then present a review of the literature focusing on dissociative phenomena as they present in violent behavior toward others and violent behavior toward the self, or auto-aggressive behavior. We conclude the chapter by offering a brief overview of psychopharmacological and psychotherapeutic remediation and suggest other, more in-depth sources.

Fine examples of the ongoing debate over intentionality and responsibility for actions in forensic settings, with particular emphases on dissociative and posttraumatic states, are presented in detail elsewhere (cf. Gilligan 1996; Wilson 1997). Furthermore, although substance abuse and dependence have sometimes been thought of as forms of "chemical dissociation" (Roesler and Dafler 1993), the interrelationship between violence and dissociative states will only be considered in cases that do not involve substance abuse.

We wish to thank Drs. N. G. Berrill and M. G. Frawley O'Dea for their support in preparing earlier drafts of the manuscript for this chapter.

Dissociation

Dissociative states exist on a continuum that ranges from normal to pathological. Davies and Frawley (1994) provided a definition for the breadth of dissociation as

> the process of severing connections between categories of mental events—between events that seem irreconcilably different, between the actual events and their affective and emotional significance, between actual events and the awareness of their cognitive significance, and finally, as in the case of severe trauma, between the actual occurrence of real events and their permanent, symbolic, verbal, mental representation. (p. 62)

Levels of Dissociation

Dissociation and dissociative states may be described at three levels: broadly, in a wide concept of dissociation; more narrowly, in terms of core dissociative features; and most narrowly, with DSM-IV (American Psychiatric Association 1994) diagnostic categories.

Wide Dissociation

A wide view of dissociation is well described by the 28 self-report items of the Dissociative Experiences Scale (DES; Bernstein and Putnam 1986), which explore the most common presentations of dissociative phenomena and describe them in simple and recognizable terms. In its mildest forms, the experience of dissociation is common to all people in the manner in which, for example, selective attention to a theme or stimulus leaves one unaware of other environmental stimuli. Familiar examples are the experience of driving a car and not remembering part or all of the trip, or absorption while watching a movie. At its most extreme, dissociation may lead to the forgetting of events or loss of recognition for familiar people or places. Screening tools such as the DES are useful in assessing *amounts* of dissociative experience but are less specific in assessing *type*. DES scores range from 0 (least) to 100 (most) and have been normed for different populations (see the discussion on dissociation in psychiatric populations later in this chapter).

Intermediate Dissociation

The intermediate level of organizing dissociative phenomena is best highlighted by Steinberg's (1995) description of the five core dissociative features and their relationship to DSM-IV dissociative disorders. These core features are amnesia, derealization, depersonalization, identity confusion, and identity alteration.

Amnesia, often considered to be the "building block" (Steinberg 1995, p. 9) on which the other dissociative symptoms rest, is characterized by gaps in memory, the sense or knowledge that time has passed but the experience cannot be recalled, individuals' realization that they have been somewhere but were "not themselves" when they went there, and a general inability to recall the frequency and duration of amnestic periods. Like the other dissociative symptoms, amnesia is highly related to histories of child abuse (Coons et al. 1988; Davies and Frawley 1994; Putnam 1985).

Derealization is the feeling of estrangement and detachment from environments that are often quite familiar to the individual. The estrangement may include both familiar places and familiar people, including family members. During flashbacks or trauma-related memories, an individual may experience the derealization of his or her current surroundings and the reliving of the past.

Depersonalization is the manner in which individuals become estranged from their sense of self, their thoughts, and even parts of their body. Aspects of an individual may take on alternative characteristics and even become represented as an internalized voice in dialogue with the normally held sense of self.

Identity confusion is "the subjective feeling of uncertainty, puzzlement, or conflict about one's own identity" (Steinberg 1995, p. 13), manifested by rapidly vacillating emotional states, and apparently contradictory self representations. Individuals with identity confusion may question the origin of their interests, persuasions, and even sexual orientation.

Identity alteration, the least common of the dissociative symptoms, is a shift in a person's identity or role, often accompanied by the assumption of a different name and marked changes in behavior and abilities. These changes, although the least common of the dissociative symptoms, are often the most obvious to other people, since they involve visible changes in a person's functioning that often influence social and professional relationships.

Narrow Dissociation

Dissociation is a highly salient, and narrowly defined, component in the following DSM-IV diagnostic categories: dissociative disorders, acute stress disorder, posttraumatic stress disorder (PTSD), and borderline personality disorder.

DSM-IV contains five dissociative disorders as Axis I diagnoses: dissociative amnesia, dissociative fugue, dissociative identity disorder (formerly multiple personality disorder), depersonalization disorder, and dissociative disorder not otherwise specified (NOS). Each of the dissociative disorders is, essentially, defined by the valence of the core dissociative features that underlie it. Furthermore, dissociative amnesia and depersonalization disorder are unique as diagnostic criteria in themselves as well as symptoms of other diagnoses. Dissociative disorder NOS describes presentations in which the core dissociative features either are not loaded in one particular direction or are loaded in an uncharacteristic manner.

Acute stress disorder and PTSD are considered to be anxiety disorders in DSM-IV and are both characterized by dissociative symptoms (Spiegel and Cardeña 1991). Although it was not officially recognized in DSM-III-R (American Psychiatric Association 1987), acute stress disorder has now been included as a separate diagnosis in DSM-IV and contains prominent dissociative and anxiety components (Koopman et al. 1995). Whereas symptoms of acute stress disorder are brief and reactive, PTSD symptoms are chronic.

Dissociative mechanisms are central processes in the genesis of PTSD (Spiegel and Cardeña 1990). These mechanisms facilitate aspects of the fragmentation of experience, encapsulation and loss of memory, and disturbances in the time sense (i.e., when past is experienced in the present) that are the hallmarks of PTSD. Diagnostic criteria for PTSD are recurrent and intrusive recollections of the traumatic event, physiological reactivity and hyperarousal to internal and external cues that symbolize or resemble an aspect of the trauma, and exaggerated startle response. Core dissociative components are amnesia, psychic numbing, feelings of detachment and estrangement, and behavioral detachment and estrangement.

DSM-IV also saw a change in the diagnostic criteria for borderline personality disorder (American Psychiatric Association 1994, p. 656) with the addition of "severe dissociative symptoms" as a ninth criterion. This addition has brought about a more than twofold increase in the number of possible diagnostic criteria combinations (from 56 to 126) for a diagnosis of borderline personality disorder and will, no doubt, cause some patients with dissociative disorders to be diagnosed with character disorders. Some clinicians (Landecker 1992) have suggested that borderline personality disorder is, in fact, a complex form of PTSD, although the issue of the role of traumatic experience in the genesis of borderline personality disorder is controversial (Soloff and Millward 1983).

Dissociation in Psychiatric Patients

The DES has been used to determine normative scores for some clinical and nonclinical populations. Supporting the premise that dissociation is a mundane psychological process, Frischholtz et al. (1990) found a DES mean score of 7.8 out of 100 for adults in the nonpsychiatric general population (N = 415). In clinical populations, Ross et al. (1994) found a mean score of 14.34 in patients with a stable diagnosis of schizophrenia (N = 83), Carlson et al. (1991) found a mean score of 30 in a population of individuals with PTSD (N = 116), and Coons et al. (1988) found a mean score of 18.2 in patients with borderline personality disorder (N = 13). Dunn et al. (1994) found a mean DES score of 14.15 in an exclusively substance-abusing population (N = 183), and Taintor and Porteus (1997) found a mean score of 27.62 in a chronically hospitalized inpatient mentally ill chemical-abusing population (N = 67), in whom severe mental illness and substance abuse were comorbid.

Past Traumatic Events in Psychiatric Patients

Psychiatric populations, compared with others, appear to have remarkably high rates of past traumatic experiences. However, these are often not explored or simply not considered in the assessment of the patient (Ross and Clark 1992). Traumatic experiences more often than not give rise to increased utilization of dissociative defenses. Violent behaviors toward self or others often dovetail with increased utilization of dissociative defenses. Therefore, understanding the rates of past traumatic events in psychiatric patients is critical to understanding the relationship between dissociation and violence.

In their study of reports of child abuse in chronic psychotic patients, Goff et al. (1991) found that 44% of the patients in their sample reported having been abused in childhood. Craine et al. (1988) found that 51% of female state hospital psychiatric patients had histories of sexual abuse, and Ross et al. (1994) found the rate of childhood histories of sexual and physical abuse to be 44.5% in a population of 83 patients with a diagnosis of schizophrenia. More recently, Briere (1997) estimated that 35%–70% of female mental health patients self-report a childhood history of sexual abuse. Sadly, these figures are large and, through replication studies, have been found to be reliable.

Case Illustration

The following case illustration is representative of some, but not all, of the key features in the relationship between violence and dissociation outlined in this chapter. Moreover, it represents an amalgam of staff observation, psychometric evaluation, and clinical interview, and thereby highlights the utility that each has in formulating a case.

Bill, who was in his early twenties, was seen on a secure care ward in a facility primarily serving the chronically mentally ill. A consultation was requested because of Bill's complaints of "forgetting," his history of childhood abuse, and the intensity and frequency of Bill's violent interactions with staff and patients, especially staff. On occasions, when Bill was placed in a seclusion room, he would wail and launch himself at the door and walls with such ferocity that the plaster walls would buckle.

Records indicate that Bill had been hospitalized over a dozen times between age 9 and the end of his teens. His most recent hospitalization had lasted for more than 2 years. The longest period that he had remained in the community since age 9 was a 3-year period when he reportedly "avoided other people as much as possible." Bill reported that he was hospitalized for various reasons during his teens, including talking to himself, fire setting, and drug and alcohol abuse. He also reported that during numerous of these hospitalizations, staff sought to "convince" him that he was suffering from multiple personality disorder and asked him to "sign confessions" agreeing with this.

Bill's parents separated when he was 5 years old. His mother obtained sole custody of Bill and his younger sibling, and he never saw his father again. When Bill was 9, his mother married her long-term boyfriend, a man who was regularly assaultive and cruel to Bill, his sibling, and their mother. One weekend, after drinking heavily while watching a sports event, the stepfather chased Bill through the house and violently sodomized him. Bill's memory for the event consists of later finding himself in a closet and seeing his hand covered with blood coming from his rectum. He relates this memory with no further detail and without affect. The following week Bill became agitated and violent toward teachers and students at school and was hospitalized in a psychiatric facility. During his teens, Bill abused alcohol and drugs and frequently ran away from home. While away, he was sexually exploited and "cared for" by men. Bill reported an increase in his violent behavior during this time. He readily acknowledged that it was he who would instigate his frequent physical fights.

When interviewed, Bill maintained that he could not control his aggression, that he would become amnestic and physiologically numb as violent interactions escalate. He did, however, acknowledge that he had come almost to "crave" the arousal and the state of hypervigilance that would precede his amnestic and numb experiences. With the interviewer, he was able to relate that he typically felt a need for stimulation and arousal, then turned to others to satisfy his need. He would annoy another person and instigate altercations, which then escalated. Meanwhile, Bill felt a rush of stimulation; he was hyperaroused, hypervigilant, and calmly aware of his surroundings. As the altercation peaked, Bill's hyperaroused state would begin to give way to a sense of numbness, and his memory for the event would fade. Just as Bill became numb, the other person would become aroused and responded to Bill's violence with violence.

Bill reported that on more than one occasion, violent episodes led to fugue states. On one occasion, Bill instigated a fight "with a man who reminded me a lot of my stepfather." He then remembered nothing more until, 2 weeks later, he found himself stepping out of a tractor-trailer at a truck stop five states away. In the intervening weeks, Bill had received medical attention, probably for injuries incurred in the fight, and had been able to travel.

Bill was evaluated by means of the Structured Clinical Interview for DSM-IV Dissociative Disorders (SCID-D; Steinberg 1994), the Structured Clinical Interview for DSM-IV Axis II Personality Disorders (SCID-II; First et al. 1996), and the DES. Results from the SCID-D indicated that Bill met criteria for an Axis I diagnosis of dissociative amnesia. His amnestic episodes were found to be severe in nature and not associated with alcohol or drugs. Mild symptoms of dissociative depersonalization and identity alteration were also detected on the SCID-D; neither was associated with alcohol or drugs. Results from the SCID-II indicated that Bill met all nine DSM-IV criteria for an Axis II diagnosis of borderline personality disorder. Bill also met diagnostic criteria for Axis II diagnoses of obsessive-compulsive personality disorder and antisocial personality disorder. Bill's overall DES score of 31.3 was high, indicating a pervasive utilization of dissociative defenses. Analysis of the factor structure of the DES revealed that in day-to-day functioning, Bill was moderately affected by dissociative amnesia and depersonalization but was severely affected by dissociative absorption and reverie.

Bill's psychometric profile teases out elements of the relationship between past traumatic events, dissociation, and violence in adulthood. Furthermore, this profile identifies everyday dissociative experiences. These are in contrast to dissociative experiences present under more extreme environmental conditions. While a diagnosis of borderline personality disorder provides a characterological description, obsessive-compulsive and antisocial features aptly describe Bill's hypervigilance, overattention to environmental cues, and ability to act impulsively and without consideration for others.

Bill readily acknowledges his pendulum-like swings across the spectrum of hyperarousal to numbness. He also elucidates the manner in which he uses other people to facilitate his craving to experience this lability. His memories are fragmented and unintegrated, yet the interpersonal matrices that he re-creates are consistent. This suggests that *what* happened is an important variable alongside *how* and *where*. Furthermore, Bill acknowledges that during the longest period in which he did not come into contact with law enforcement or mental health authorities he avoided other people.

Violence and Dissociation

Dysregulation, Repetition, and Violence: The Interpersonal Dimension

After a history of systemic psychological insult, the emotional spectrum may often appear as an affective Möbius strip. Individuals experiencing extreme states of psychic numbing may suddenly become physiologically and behaviorally hyperaroused. The inverse is also true, whereby a state of hyperarousal may have led to a state of psychic numbness.

The inability to modulate physiological arousal or overwhelming psychic experience has a cascade of effects on both the individual's behavior and his or her interpersonal relations. The behavioral "spillovers" of affects that cannot be regulated cause impairment in social functioning as a result of hypervigilance, increased attention to internal stimuli, and, in some cases, a tendency to instigate or trigger the environment in such a way that a past traumatic event may be reenacted (van der Kolk and Greenberg 1987). Moreover, the roles of perpetrator and victim become confused in these violent interpersonal dyads.

Chronic alterations in the central nervous system have been noted as a result of hyperarousal after traumatic exposure (Russ 1992; van der Kolk et al. 1985). Elevated plasma endorphin levels have been reported as a response to physiological stress (Bortz et al. 1981; Colt et al. 1981), surgery (Cohen et al. 1982), and gambling (Blaszczynski et al. 1984). As a result, certain individuals may become "addicted" not to a traumatic environment, but to the rush of endogenous opioids that it can cause (van der Kolk 1989). They may be bent on re-creating an endogenous opioid rush interpersonally.

As Bach-y-Rita and Veno (1974) studied incarcerated men who were routinely violent toward other people, they found that these same perpetrators would self-mutilate when isolated from others. Others (like Bill) would precipitate/instigate violence toward themselves by stimulating and hyperarousing others. They became stimulated and hyperaroused themselves and would then be beaten into a state of opioid-induced psychic numbness. This parsing of the dissociative mechanisms of hyperarousal and psychic numbing into each member of a dyad has also been observed in couples therapy with patients with combat-related PTSD (Johnson et al. 1995) and in transference and countertransference states in psychotherapy (Frawley O'Dea 1997; Howell 1996), in which one member of the dyad is hyperaroused and the other is numb.

Encapsulation, Engraving of Memory, and Violence

Neuroimaging studies (Rauch et al. 1996) have shown that the processing of posttraumatic events involves nonverbal areas of the brain, such as the temporal lobe and limbic system. Moreover, the studies show a "turning off" of verbal processing regions, particularly Wernicke's and Broca's areas, such as is found in alexithymia.

Memory is an active and constructive process (van der Kolk and van der Hart 1991). However, general systemic impingement under stressful conditions may impair hippocampal function as well as give rise to somatosensory and iconic sensation, behavioral reenactment, and flashbacks (Brett and Ostroff 1985). Concurrent, intense autonomic activation interferes with behavioral processing and the engraving of memory (van der Kolk and van der Hart 1991). For example, Wilkinson (1983) found that 27% of the survivors of the Hyatt Regency skywalk collapse had memory difficulties.

Without recourse to normal emotional expression and modulation through the language centers and their frontal lobe motoric corollaries, highly charged affective states remain as encapsulated, nonverbal, visceral experiences. These experiences ultimately kindle affect storms and implicit, uncensored action through an oblique connection between affect and action (van der Kolk and van der Hart 1991). This dissociation, which is a response to what is unknown or intangible, has been described in the violence literature on automatic thinking and psychological blow automatism (Febbo et al. 1993–1994), and in multiple reports of defendants who are amnestic to their violent crime (Taylor and Kopelman 1984).

States of hyperarousal with material moving out of conscious awareness clearly involve the phenomenological experience of dissociation, but they do not necessarily imply systemic decompensation. For example, in a striking investigation of dissociation and ego organization, Salley and Teiling (1984) describe the Rorschach data of a Vietnam combat veteran with episodic dissociated rage attacks that suggest near neurotic levels of ego functioning despite massively dissociated outbursts. This dissociation is at times simple amnesia and at other times a derealization of the environment or depersonalization of self. As investigators have increasingly clarified the dissociative disorders, some have published attempts to understand violent dissociative states, mainly in the forensic literature.

Dissociation and Loss of Self-Control: Neurobiological Rudiments

Loss of self-control and dissociation may have more than merely phenomenological similarities. As the understanding of the neurobiological pathways underlying impulsivity, aggression, dissociation, and trauma has advanced, some apparent etiologic similarities may be noted. One important similarity that has emerged is that serotonergic and noradrenergic mechanisms have been implicated in both loss of self-control and dissociation. This may provide clues for psychopharmacological remediation.

The literature exploring the neurobiology of violence, impulsivity, and aggression, broadly summarized by Volavka (1995), suggests a relationship between serotonergic pathways and more prosocial action, and a relationship between noradrenergic pathways and more antisocial action. Similarly, van der Kolk and Saporta (1991) and van der Kolk (1996), in their reviews, found that the literature suggests that the efficacies of the ascending serotonergic and cholinergic mechanisms are disrupted in states of dissociation and trauma, leading to a breakdown in modulation between the serotonergic and noradrenergic mechanisms and a net increase in behavior that is impulsive and not under the individual's control.

Review of the Literature

Dissociative Phenomena and Outward Aggression

Although the relationship between violence and dissociation appears, in many instances, to be an intuitive one, the literature relating the two is limited. Ideally, the relationship between these two variables would best be explored in large community samples such as those in the

Epidemiologic Catchment Area studies, but such studies have not explored dissociation. Those studies that are available tend to be skewed toward populations that are hypothesized to have high rates of dissociation, such as specific psychiatric populations, or populations in which dissociative phenomena could usefully account for variations between subgroups, such as in the criminal justice system. Moreover, some studies rely on "stand-in" variables for dissociation—that is, variables that are significantly related to dissociation, such as child abuse, PTSD, and Axis II pathology such as borderline personality disorder.

In the following review of the dissociation literature as it pertains to outwardly directed violence, we first discuss the relationship between histories of abuse and consequent dissociation and violent crime. We then provide a more general review of dissociation and violence in the criminal justice system and conclude with a focus on externally oriented violence and dissociation in psychiatric patients.

Dissociation, Past Traumatic Events, and Criminality

A history of childhood victimization not only predicts elevated levels of dissociative phenomena but also delinquent behavior (Alfaro 1978; Gutierres and Reich 1981; Kratcoski 1982), adult antisocial personality disorder (Luntz and Widom 1994), and violent criminal behavior (Curtis 1963; Garbarino and Gilliam 1980; Lewis 1993; Tarter et al. 1984; Widom 1989a, 1989b). Kluft (1987) found that up to 16% of mothers with extreme dissociative presentations, who had themselves been abused, abused one or more of their own children. Clearly, a relationship exists between past abuse and violence.

Rivera and Widom (1990) assessed the long-term criminal consequences of officially documented childhood abuse, including physical abuse, sexual abuse, and neglect, through an examination of official criminal histories in adulthood. The experimental group consisted of 908 individuals who had been victims of child abuse and whose cases were processed through the courts between 1967 and 1971. A matched sample of individuals ($n = 667$) with no official record of abuse as children was then selected. The control sample was carefully matched for age, ethnicity, gender, and socioeconomic status. Moreover, the control sample was selected from the same neighborhoods as the experimental sample. Although past comparisons of adult arrest rates suggested a significantly increased rate of arrest for any crime for those with histories of early childhood victimization (Widom 1989a), these data clearly showed an increased rate of violent offending in adulthood, particularly for males. In a later study, Widom and Ames (1994) showed that victims of childhood sexual abuse are at higher risk for arrest for perpetration of adult sex crimes than are control subjects. There was also among males a suggestion of an association between a history of childhood physical abuse and neglect and perpetration of adult sex crimes.

Another researcher who has greatly contributed to the literature in this area, D. Otnow Lewis (1993), has suggested that childhood maltreatment in the form of abuse or neglect exacerbates preexisting psychological and psychobiological vulnerabilities. According to Lewis, maltreatment early in life has a cascade of effects, including later increased impulsivity and irritability, hypervigilance and paranoia, diminished judgment and verbal competence, and dampening of the recognition of pain in self and others. Dissociation is pervasive in this profile.

Dissociation and Violence in the Criminal Justice System

Patients who have come into contact with the criminal justice system have also prompted a greater understanding of the role of dissociation in violence. For example, one diagnostic revision that was proposed for DSM-III-R was inclusion of a beserker/blind rage syndrome in the dissociative disorders (Simon 1987). In this proposed epiphenomenon, violent dissociated rage attacks are characterized by 1) intense violent reaction to insult with loss of control of violent impulses, 2) amnesia during the period of violence, 3) abnormal fluctuations in strength, and 4) specific, target-oriented violence. All four of these criteria incorporate a dissociative function, be it neurobiological (dysregulation and dyscontrol), somatic (fluctuation in physical strength), or psychic (an ability to selectively focus on specific stimuli).

As noted earlier in this chapter, dissociated blind rage is often accompanied by amnesia. Pollock (1996), in describing the relationship between violence and dissociative amnesia in sexually abused women who committed violent offenses against their partners in intimate relationships, reported amnestic states before, during, and after their violent acts. In a more extreme presentation, Febbo et al. (1993–1994) reported a case of dissociated amnesia and "Psychological Blow Automatism" in which a 51-year-old woman shot and killed her husband at close range. In this instance the presence of dissociated, automatic, and involuntary actions was upheld by the courts in a case in which the defendant was simultaneously considered "sane."

Dissociative Amnesia

Amnesia for violent acts is not an uncommon criminal defense. It is claimed by as many as 30%–40% of perpetrators in homicide cases (Kopelman 1987a, 1987b) and is a recent focus of the dissociation literature. The science of distinguishing true from malingering dissociative amnesia is not well advanced (Kluft 1994; Kopelman 1987b). However, Parwatikar et al. (1985), in exploring the detection of malingered amnesia in accused murderers, noted that the defendant who malingers and convinces a psychiatrist that he or she has amnesia has won a Pyrrhic victory, because a court will rarely find a defendant incompetent to stand trial because of amnesia alone.

Taylor and Kopelman (1984) studied 212 men on custodial remand for violent and nonviolent crimes in which 19 men claimed amnesia for their offense. In these cases the amnesia was considered to have no legal implications for the individual's criminal defense and, thereby, to have no secondary gain. Of the sample of 19 amnesic individuals, all had committed a violent crime: 9 committed murder or manslaughter, 6 personal violence or arson, and 4 criminal damage. All 19 qualified for a psychiatric diagnosis: 7 for schizophrenia, 4 for depressive illness, and 8 for alcoholism or serious substance abuse.

As part of the same study, Taylor and Kopelman (1984) included a violence rating (Gunn and Bonn 1971; Gunn and Robertson 1976), which was used to assess the level of violence of each individual's offense, and the Beck Depression Inventory (Beck et al. 1961) to assess the offenders. They found that offenses of the amnestic group were significantly more violent. Also, the amnestic offenders had significantly higher depression ratings than the nonamnestic offenders. The authors considered organic and substance-induced states as variables that could have distinguished amnesic and nonamnesic groups but favored psychological defense mechanisms. The amnesic group was not distinguishable from the nonamnesic group on tests of orientation, memory, and cerebral function. Moreover, the proportion of alcoholic or substance-abusing men who committed violent crimes in the amnesic group was equal to the proportion of alcoholic or substance-abusing men who had a memory for their violent acts. Intoxication at the time of the violent act was not a significant factor for either group.

Dissociation and Aggression in a Psychiatric Inpatient Cohort

Quimby and Putnam (1991) assessed the relationship between dissociative symptoms and aggression in a cohort of 70 psychiatric inpatients.

Forty-three of these patients were male, and 27 were female. In addition to the DES, this study utilized the Modified Overt Aggression Scale (MOAS; Kay et al. 1988) and a parallel sexual aggression scale measuring behaviors from molestation to rape. The MOAS, and its predecessor, the Overt Aggression Scale (OAS; Yudofsky et al. 1986), are widely used to identify four types of aggression: verbal, physical against self, physical against others, and physical aggression against objects. There are four degrees of severity for each aggressive type, with each degree being defined by anchor points. Both the MOAS and the sexual aggression scale use a psychiatric treatment team's evaluations of patients' overt aggressive behavior. Of the sample in this study, 30% scored 30 or higher on the DES, and 14.3% scored over 45.

The results indicate a significant relationship between overt aggression and dissociation across gender. However, although results indicated a significant relationship between high dissociation and overt aggression in the male population, no significant relationship was found between these variables in the female population. Dissociation and aggression in males were more often associated with aggression toward others, property damage, and sexual aggression, while dissociation in females was more often related to self-directed aggression and sexual aggression.

Dissociative Phenomena and Auto-Aggression

The literature pertaining to self-directed violence and dissociation is even more limited than the literature pertaining to outwardly directed violence and dissociation. The clearest evidence is the lack of data regarding suicide and dissociation. Three exceptions are the works of Ross and Norton (1989) and Kluft (1994), which deal exclusively with suicide attempts in patients diagnosed with multiple personality disorder/dissociative identity disorder, and the work of Freeman et al. (1995), whose sample was drawn from a population with PTSD. Expanding the topic of auto-aggression to nonlethal violent self-directed acts, Coons and Milstein (1990) explored the relationship between dissociative disorders and less serious auto-aggression, and Zlotnick et al. (1996) compared self-mutilating patients on a women's psychiatric unit with female patients without a history of self-mutilation.

Dissociation and Suicidal Behavior

Ross and Norton (1989) found that 85.4% of a sample of 167 patients with multiple personality disorder/dissociative identity disorder who attempted suicide did so by overdosing. Also, within this sample, 68.7% were found to have inflicted cigarette burns or committed other self-mutilating acts, and 60.4% had slashed their wrists. Kluft (1994) found that 65% of a sample of 40 patients with multiple personality disorder/ dissociative identity disorder had made a serious suicide attempt, and one patient had completed suicide.

Freeman et al. (1995) compared ratings for a group of 14 patients with a history of suicide attempts with those for 16 patients without such a history. Although significant between-group differences were not found for ratings from the PTSD-I (PTSD Interview), Michigan Alcoholism Screening Test, Drug Abuse Screening Test, and Combat Exposure Scale, scores on the DES were significantly higher in the group with a history of suicide attempts. Moreover, those patients in the group without a history of suicide attempts tended to consider or take into account the potential lethality of their weapons more than did the members of the group with a history of suicide.

Dissociation and Nonlethal Auto-Aggression

What remains to be described in the literature on auto-aggression are violent behaviors that are typically impulsive, chronic, and repetitive, without accompanying suicidal ideation and of low lethality, involving multiple methods of self-injury (Pattison and Kahan 1983; Walsh and Rosen 1988). Wrist cutting may be considered a prototypical self-mutilating behavior; however, burning, self-hitting, and severe self-mutilation (cf. Gardner and Cowdry 1985) are also subsumed in the category of self-destructive acts.

Coons and Milstein (1990) have attempted to identify the relationship between particular dissociative disorders and violence toward the self. Although they have not generated specific data regarding dissociative derealization and dissociative disorder NOS, their data indicate histories of self-directed violence in 29% of patients with dissociative amnesia, 20% of patients in dissociative fugue states (Coons and Milstein 1992), and 48% of patients with dissociative identity disorder.

Further evidence of the role of dissociation in auto-aggression has been provided by Zlotnick et al. (1996), who studied 103 self-mutilating patients on a women's psychiatric unit and compared them with 45 patients with no history of self-mutilation. When the cohort was screened with the DES, the self-mutilating group was found to have significantly higher rates of dissociation. Moreover, significantly higher rates of alexithymia, as measured by the Toronto Alexithymia Scale, were also found in the self-mutilating group. In conclusion, rates of dissociation and level of alexithymia were both found to be positively correlated with the number of self-injurious acts that patients committed. As noted earlier, alexithymia, or the inability to verbalize experience, may be related to the common dissociative posttraumatic response in which temporal lobe processing gains dominance and experiences are often encapsulated in a nonverbal form.

The dissociation literature often relates auto-aggression to the modulation of dissociative depersonalization and dissociative derealization. Violence against the self, in the form of self-mutilation, has been related to the modulation of states of dissociative depersonalization (Coons and Milstein 1990; Kluft 1994; Waltzer 1968). States of depersonalization involve a fundamental shifting of the individual's sense of who he or she is. One way to combat the increased experience of depersonalization is through auto-aggression. In auto-aggressive states, which often go "unfelt," self-mutilating individuals ground themselves by making the connection between the experience of who they are and the experience of their body hypersalient, thereby diminishing or eradicating their loss of identity.

Another dissociative component in self-directed violence is the control or diminution of pain. In this context, dissociative derealization appears to allow the patient not to experience the pain involved in self-injurious behaviors. Russ et al. (1993) used the DES to screen a population of self-mutilating female patients with borderline personality disorder. The authors found that the rates of dissociation were significantly higher in those subjects who did not experience their pain while injuring themselves than in those who reported experiencing the pain of their self-mutilation.

Remediation

As noted earlier in this chapter, a careful interview and case history are essential in working with patients with the potential for violence and dissociation, especially since dissociating individuals who commit particularly severe violent acts experience amnesia of some kind. Although there is a paucity of literature relating to psychopharmacological interventions, a wider body of literature exists for psychotherapeutic treatments.

Psychopharmacological

Until recently, psychopharmacological remediation of dissociative states was not possible. Instead, clinicians were required to treat the secondary symptoms of dissociation, including violence.

Kluft (1984) first noted the use of carbamazepine in the control of rapidly fluctuating dissociation. This medication was reported to reduce intrusive symptoms (Lipper et al. 1986) and aggressive outbursts (Wolf et al. 1988) in combat veterans with PTSD. Carbamazepine has also been used effectively in decreasing episodic violence in patients with dissociative disorders and increasing control of dissociation (Coons 1992; Fichtner et al. 1990).

Van der Kolk et al. (1994) assessed the efficacy of fluoxetine in PTSD in a study, using, among other measures, a hostility inventory and the DES. They found a significant decrease in all measures (most notably in the arousal and numbing symptom categories) for fluoxetine compared with placebo. They suggested that serotonin reuptake inhibitors may effectively modulate aggressive behavior in chronically dissociating patients. It has also been suggested (Davidson and van der Kolk 1996; Saporta and Case 1991) that hallucination and delusions accompanying flashbacks and dissociated states may also diminish with low doses of antipsychotic medication.

Psychotherapeutic

The primary task of the therapeutic process is to link thought and feeling in order to reintegrate experiences that can be consciously tolerated by the patient. In treating violent dissociating patients, the therapist must emphasize increased insight into the patient's behavioral and physiological reactions to environmental stimuli as well as containment of responses to internal and external cues (Grame 1993). Groups for violent patients who dissociate can help patients hear about behaviors that mirror their own experience and bring the interpersonal nature of these behaviors into focus in their individual treatments.

As noted earlier, the laying down of memory may be affected by extreme environmental concomitants. At times this may lead to partial memories or to full memories that are kaleidoscopic and not easily integrated. It is vitally important that the therapist make a detailed assessment, because *where* the experience occurred may be more informative and available than an understanding of *what* actually occurred. This is especially important when a patient manipulates his or her interpersonal experiences in order to re-create familiar aspects of past experiences.

Descriptions of psychotherapeutic treatment approaches to dissociative phenomena are readily available in the literature. Treatments may be selected according to the nature of the patient presentation, the therapeutic orientation of the clinician, and the level of functioning of the patient. Fine examples of treatment approaches for these populations may be found elsewhere (e.g., Allen and Smith 1995; Davies and Frawley 1994; Everly and Lating 1995; Pollock 1996; van der Kolk et al. 1996).

Conclusion

The relationship between violence and dissociation is complex, with multiple determinants. Although the relationship has been relatively understudied, dissociation should be a prominent consideration in the aftermath of violence. Clearly, dissociative states create an environment in which violent and impulsive acts are more likely. Fortunately, the more recent focus on dissociative processes and their relationship with violence has been facilitated by an advance in our understanding of dissociative phenomena and greater clarity in their definition. As the inquiry gains in breadth and depth, a clearer picture of the biological, psychological, and social backdrop to dissociation and violence should emerge.

There remains a need for further study of these interrelationships, including clarification of the role of past traumatic events, exploration of potential biochemical markers, elaboration of psychological assessment (including the assessment of malingering), and development and refinement of treatment approaches. It should be noted that these tasks have taken on an added measure of complexity, given the reemergence of traditional disputes over "hysterical" states and the pitfalls of the debate over "false" versus "recovered" memories. Rather than deterring further inquiry, these challenges should emphasize the need for reliability and validity in future research.

References

Alfaro J: Child Abuse and Subsequent Delinquent Behavior. New York, Select Committee on Child Abuse, 1978

Allen JG, Smith WH (eds): Diagnosis and Treatment of Dissociative Disorders. Northvale, NJ, Jason Aronson, 1995

American Psychiatric Association: Diagnostic and Statistical Manual of Mental Disorders, 3rd Edition, Revised. Washington, DC, American Psychiatric Association, 1987

American Psychiatric Association: Diagnostic and Statistical Manual of Mental Disorders, 4th Edition. Washington, DC, American Psychiatric Association, 1994

Bach-y-Rita G, Veno A: Habitual violence: a profile of 62 men. Am J Psychiatry 131:1015–1017, 1974

Beck AT, Ward CH, Mendelson M, et al: An inventory for measuring depression. Arch Gen Psychiatry 4:561–571, 1961

Bernstein EM, Putnam FW: Development, reliability, and validity of a dissociation scale. J Nerv Ment Dis 174:727–735, 1986

Blaszczynski AP, Winter SW, McConaghy X: Plasma endorphin levels in pathological gambling. Paper presented at the Sixth Annual Conference on Gambling and Risk Taking, Atlantic City, NJ, 1984

Bortz WM, Angevin P, Mefford IN, et al: Catecholamines, dopamine, and endorphin levels during extreme exercise. N Engl J Med 305:466–469, 1981

Brett EA, Ostroff R: Imagery and post-traumatic stress disorder: an overview. Am J Psychiatry 142:417–424, 1985

Briere J: Psychological Assessment of Adult Posttraumatic States. Washington, DC, American Psychological Association, 1997

Carlson EB, Putnam FW, Ross CA, et al: Factor analysis of the Dissociative Experiences Scale: a multicenter study. Paper presented at the Eighth International Conference on Multiple Personality and Dissociative States, Chicago, IL, 1991

Cohen MR, Pichas D, Dubois M, et al: Stress induced plasma beta endorphin immunoreactivity may predict postoperative morphine usage. Psychiatry Res 6:7–12, 1982

Colt EW, Wardlaw SL, Frantz AG: The effect of running on plasma beta endorphin. Life Sci 28:1637–1640, 1981

Coons PM: The use of carbamazepine for episodic violence in multiple personality disorder and dissociative disorder not otherwise specified: two additional cases. Biol Psychiatry 32:717–720, 1992

Coons PM, Milstein V: Self mutilation associated with dissociative disorders. Dissociation 3:81–87, 1990

Coons PM, Milstein V: Psychogenic amnesia: a clinical study of 50 cases. Dissociation 5:73–79, 1992

Coons PM, Bowman ES, Milstein V: Multiple personality disorder: a clinical investigation of 50 cases. J Nerv Ment Dis 176:519–527, 1988

Craine LS, Henson CH, Colliver JA, et al: Prevalence of a history of sexual abuse among female psychiatric patients in a state hospital system. Hospital and Community Psychiatry 39:300–304, 1988

Curtis GC: Violence breeds violence—perhaps? Am J Psychiatry 120: 386–387, 1963

Davidson JRT, van der Kolk BA: The psychopharmacological treatment of posttraumatic stress disorder, in Traumatic Stress. Edited by van der Kolk BA, McFarlane AC, Weisaeth L. New York, Guilford, 1996, pp 242–260

Davies J, Frawley MG: The Psychodynamic Treatment of Adult Survivors of Childhood Sexual Abuse. New York, Basic Books, 1994

Dunn GE, Ryan JJ, Paolo AM: A principal components analysis of the Dissociative Experiences Scale in a substance abuse population. J Clin Psychol 50:936–940, 1994

Everly GS, Lating JM (eds): Psychotraumatology: Key Papers and Core Concepts in Post-traumatic Stress. New York, Plenum, 1995

Febbo S, Hardy F, Finlay-Jones R: Dissociation and psychological blow automatism in Australia. Int J Ment Health 22:39–59, 1993–1994

Fichtner CG, Kuhlman DT, Gruenfeld MJ, et al: Decreased episodic violence and increased control of dissociation in a carbamazepine treated case of multiple personality. Biol Psychiatry 27:1045–1052, 1990

First MB, Gibbon M, Spitzer RL, et al: User's Guide for the Structured Clinical Interview for DSM-IV Axis II Personality Disorders (SCID-II, Version 2.0, July 1996 Final Version). New York, New York State Psychiatric Institute, 1996

Frawley O'Dea MG: Who's doing what to whom? Supervision and sexual abuse. Contemporary Psychoanalysis 33:5–18, 1997

Freeman TW, Keesee N, Thornton C, et al: Dissociative symptoms in posttraumatic stress disorder subjects with a history of suicide attempts. J Nerv Ment Dis 183:664–666, 1995

Frischholtz EJ, Brown BG, Sachs RG: The Dissociative Experiences Scale: further replication and validation. Dissociation 3:151–153, 1990

Garbarino J, Gilliam G: Understanding Abusive Families. Lexington, MA, Lexington Books, 1980

Gardner DL, Cowdry RW: Suicidal and parasuicidal behavior in borderline personality disorder. Psychiatr Clin North Am 8:389–403, 1985

Gilligan J: Violence: Our Deadly Epidemic and Its Causes. New York, Putnam, 1996

Goff DC, Brotman AW, Kindlon D, et al: Self reports of childhood abuse in chronically psychotic patients. Psychiatry Res 37:73–80, 1991

Grame CJ: Internal containment in the treatment of patients with dissociative disorders. Bull Menninger Clin 57:355–361, 1993

Gunn J, Bonn J: Criminality and violence in epileptic prisoners. Br J Psychiatry 118:337–343, 1971

Gunn J, Robertson G: Drawing a criminal profile. British Journal of Criminology 16:156–160, 1976

Gutierres S, Reich JA: A developmental perspective on runaway behavior: its relationship to child abuse. Child Welfare 60:89–94, 1981

Howell E: Dissociation in masochism and psychopathic sadism. Contemporary Psychoanalysis 32:427–453, 1996

Johnson DR, Feldman S, Lubin H: Critical interaction therapy: couples therapy in combat-related post traumatic stress disorder. Family Process 34:401–412, 1995

Kay SR, Wolkenfeld F, Murrill LM: Profiles of aggression among psychiatric patients. J Nerv Ment Dis 176:539–546, 1988

Kluft RP: Aspects of the treatment of multiple personality disorder. Psychiatric Annals 14:51–55, 1984

Kluft RP: The parental fitness of mothers with multiple personality disorder: a preliminary study. Child Abuse Negl 11:272–280, 1987

Kluft RP: Dissociative disorders, in Handbook of Aggressive and Destructive Behavior in Psychiatric Patients. Edited by Hersen M, Ammerman RT, Sisson LA. New York, Plenum, 1994, pp 237–259

Koopman C, Classen C, Cardeña E, et al: When disaster strikes, acute stress disorder may follow. Journal of Traumatic Stress 8:29–46, 1995

Kopelman MD: Amnesia: organic and psychogenic. Br J Psychiatry 150:428–442, 1987a

Kopelman MD: Crime and amnesia: a review. Behavioral Sciences and the Law 5:323–342, 1987b

Kratcoski PC: Child abuse and violence against the family. Child Welfare 61:435–444, 1982

Landecker H: The role of childhood sexual trauma in the etiology of borderline personality disorder: considerations for diagnosis and treatment. Psychotherapy 29:234–242, 1992

Lewis DO: From abuse to violence: psychophysiological consequences of maltreatment. Annual Progress in Child Psychiatry and Child Development :507–527, 1993

Lipper S, Davidson JRT, Grady TA, et al: Preliminary study of carbamazepine in post-traumatic stress disorder. Psychosomatics 27:849–853, 1986

Luntz BK, Widom CS: Antisocial personality disorder in abused and neglected children grown up. Am J Psychiatry 151:670–674, 1994

Parwatikar SD, Holcomb WR, Menninger KA: The detection of malingered amnesia in accused murderers. Bull Am Acad Psychiatry Law 13:97–103, 1985

Pattison EM, Kahan T: The deliberate self-harm syndrome. Am J Psychiatry 140:867–872, 1983

Pollock PH: Clinical issues in the cognitive analytic therapy of sexually abused women who commit violent offences against their partners. Br J Med Psychol 69:117–127, 1996

Putnam FW Jr: Dissociation as a response to extreme trauma, in Childhood Antecedents of Multiple Personality. Edited by Kluft RP. Washington, DC, American Psychiatric Press, 1985, pp 65–97

Quimby LG, Putnam FW Jr: Dissociative symptoms and aggression in a state mental hospital. Dissociation 4:21–24, 1991

Rauch SL, van der Kolk BA, Fisler RE, et al: A symptom provocation study of posttraumatic stress disorder using positron emission tomography and script-driven imagery. Arch Gen Psychiatry 53:380–387, 1996

Rivera B, Widom CS: Childhood victimization and violent offending. Violence and Victims 5:19–35, 1990

Roesler TA, Dafler CE: Chemical dissociation in adults sexually victimized as children: alcohol and drug use in adult survivors. J Subst Abuse Treat 10:537–543, 1993

Ross CA, Clark P: Assessment of childhood trauma and dissociation in an emergency department. Dissociation 5:163–165, 1992

Ross CA, Norton G: Suicide and parasuicide in multiple personality disorder. Psychiatry 52:365–371, 1989

Ross CA, Anderson G, Clark P: Childhood abuse and the positive symptoms of schizophrenia. Hospital and Community Psychiatry 45:489–491, 1994

Russ MJ: Self-injurious behavior in patients with borderline personality disorder: biological perspectives. J Personal Disord 6:64–81, 1992

Russ MJ, Shearin EN, Clarkin JF, et al: Subtypes of self-injurious patients with borderline personality disorder. Am J Psychiatry 150:1869–1871, 1993

Salley RD, Teiling PA: Dissociated rage attacks in a Vietnam veteran: a Rorschach study. J Pers Assess 48:98–104, 1984

Saporta JA, Case J: The role of medication in treating adult survivors of childhood trauma, in Treating Adult Survivors of Incest. Edited by Paddison P. Washington, DC, American Psychiatric Press, 1991, pp 101–134

Simon A: The Berserker/Blind Rage Syndrome as a potentially new diagnostic category for the DSM III. Psychol Rep 60:131–135, 1987

Soloff PH, Millward JW: Developmental histories of borderline patients. Compr Psychiatry 24:574–588, 1983

Spiegel D, Cardeña E: Dissociative mechanisms in posttraumatic stress disorder, in Posttraumatic Stress Disorder: Etiology, Phenomenology, and Treatment. Edited by Wolf M, Mosnaim A. Washington, DC, American Psychiatric Press, 1990, pp 22–34

Spiegel D, Cardeña E: Disintegrated experience: the dissociative disorders revisited. J Abnorm Psychol 100:366–378, 1991

Steinberg M: Structured Clinical Interview for DSM-IV Dissociative Disorders (SCID-D), Revised. Washington, DC, American Psychiatric Press, 1994

Steinberg M: Handbook for the Assessment of Dissociation: A Clinical Guide. Washington, DC, American Psychiatric Press, 1995

Taintor Z, Porteus AJ: A psychometric profile of dissociative phenomena in chronically hospitalized mentally ill chemically abusing (MICA) inpatients: preliminary data. Paper presented at the 150th annual meeting of the American Psychiatric Association. San Diego, CA, May 1997

Tarter RE, Hegedus AM, Winsten NE, et al: Neuropsychological, personality, and familial characteristics of physically abused delinquents. Journal of the American Academy of Child Psychiatry 23: 668–674, 1984

Taylor PJ, Kopelman MD: Amnesia for criminal offences. Psychol Med 14:581–588, 1984

van der Kolk BA: The compulsion to repeat the trauma: re-enactment, re-victimization, and masochism. Psychiatr Clin North Am 12:389–411, 1989

van der Kolk BA: The body keeps score: approaches to the psychobiology of posttraumatic stress disorder, in Traumatic Stress. Edited by van der Kolk BA, McFarlane AC, Weisaeth L. New York, Guilford, 1996, pp 214–241

van der Kolk BA, Greenberg MS: The psychobiology of the trauma response: hyperarousal, constriction, and addiction to traumatic reexposure, in Psychological Trauma. Edited by van der Kolk BA. Washington, DC, American Psychiatric Press, 1987, pp 63–87

van der Kolk BA, Saporta J: The biological response to psychic trauma: mechanisms and treatment of intrusion and numbing. Anxiety Research 4:199–212, 1991

van der Kolk BA, van der Hart O: The intrusive past: the flexibility of memory and the engraving of trauma. American Imago 48:425–454, 1991

van der Kolk BA, Greenberg MS, Boyd H, et al: Inescapable shock, neurotransmitters and addiction to trauma: towards a psychobiology of post traumatic stress. Biol Psychiatry 20:314–325, 1985

van der Kolk BA, Dreyfuss D, Michaels M, et al: Fluoxetine in posttraumatic stress disorder. J Clin Psychiatry 55:517–522, 1994

van der Kolk BA, McFarlane AC, Weisaeth L (eds): Traumatic Stress. New York, Guilford, 1996

Volavka J: Neurobiology of Violence. Washington, DC, American Psychiatric Press, 1995

Walsh BW, Rosen PM: Self Mutilation—Theory, Research, and Treatment. New York, Guilford, 1988

Waltzer H: Depersonalization and self-destruction. Am J Psychiatry 42: 195–206, 1968

Widom CS: Child abuse, neglect, and adult behavior: research design and findings on criminality, violence, and child abuse. Am J Orthopsychiatry 59:355–367, 1989a

Widom CS: Does violence beget violence? A critical examination of the literature. Psychol Bull 106:3–28, 1989b

Widom CS, Ames MA: Criminal consequences of childhood sexual victimization. Child Abuse Negl 18:303–318, 1994

Wilkinson CB: Aftermath of a disaster: the collapse of the Hyatt Regency Hotel skywalk. Am J Psychiatry 140:1134–1143, 1983

Wilson JQ: Mitigating Circumstances: Law, Science and Personal Responsibility. New York, Basic Books, 1997

Wolf ME, Atavi A, Mosnaim AD: Posttraumatic stress disorder in Vietnam veterans: clinical and EEG findings, possible therapeutic effects of carbamazepine. Biol Psychiatry 23:642–644, 1988

Yudofsky SC, Silver JM, Jackson W: The Overt Aggression Scale for the objective rating of verbal and physical aggression. Am J Psychiatry 143:35–39, 1986

Zlotnick C, Shea MT, Pearlstein T, et al: The relationship between dissociative symptoms, alexithymia, impulsivity, sexual abuse, and self mutilation. Compr Psychiatry 37:12–16, 1996

CHAPTER 8

Impulse Control: Integrative Aspects

Menahem Krakowski, M.D., Ph.D.

Psychiatrists are often called on to judge impulse control or impulsivity. This happens when they treat a depressed and potentially suicidal patient, when they interview a patient who threatens an employer or a former spouse, when they decide if a mentally ill patient needs involuntary commitment, or when they assign DSM-IV diagnoses (American Psychiatric Association 1994). Impulsivity is a defining trait of borderline and antisocial personality disorders as well as the group of impulse-control disorders not elsewhere classified. Many other patients have impulse-control problems, including those with mania, schizophrenia, and dementias. Although impulsivity plays a major role in clinical decisions (Segal et al. 1988), for many it is a poorly defined and colloquial term, unlike, for example, psychosis.

In this chapter I attempt to develop an understanding of the meaning of impulsivity by considering how impulse control develops and how it is regulated and disturbed by biological factors and life experiences. I review the impressive literature documenting the association between serotonin and impulsivity and propose how that literature can illuminate the meaning of impulsivity in clinical contexts. To broaden our understanding of impulse control, I conclude the chapter by considering the psychological, social, and biological processes and the complex interplay between them.

Definitions of Impulse and Impulsivity

The terms *impulse* and *impulsive* must be distinguished to minimize confusion, as should the different meanings of impulsive. The term

This work was supported by grant MH-45454 from the National Institute of Mental Health.

impulse is closely linked to the concept of instinct and drive. An impulse is an underlying instinctive urge that incites action. Impulses vary in prevalence and acceptability. Some, like sexual ones, are universal and serve obvious biological function; others, such as impulses to set fires (pyromania) or steal in the absence of any monetary gain (kleptomania), are much more difficult to account for. Aggressive impulses are prevalent in nonhuman species, in which they serve a variety of well-defined functions. In human beings, however, they have less distinct functions and are thoroughly modified through socialization.

This emphasis on instinct and drive has been maintained in psychoanalytic literature, where the term *impulsive* is used interchangeably with *instinctive* (Hinsie and Campbell 1960). In general psychiatry, *impulsive* often denotes a failure to resist an impulse or urge. However, the term is frequently used to characterize quick and immediate responsivity—a tendency to respond without reflection (H. Murray 1938). Emphasis is placed on the *mechanism* of action, which bypasses or shortcuts the usual "pathways," and not its *derivation* in instinctual drives.

This ambiguity in definition may lead to some confusion. *Impulsive* can be used to describe the failure to resist an impulse even when considerable planning and premeditation are involved. This is best illustrated by impulse-control disorders, in which the main criterion is "failure to resist an impulse, drive, or temptation to perform an act that is harmful to the person or to others" (American Psychiatric Association 1994, p. 609). For example, patients with pyromania have an irresistible impulse to set fires; acting on the impulse relieves the tension they experience. This disorder has often been described as impulsive, although fire setting requires considerable advance planning and preparation and is certainly not undertaken rapidly. It is classified by certain authors as the prototype of an "impulsive" crime (Virkkunen et al. 1987), whereas others classify it among the least impulsive crimes (Heilbrun 1979).

Factors Affecting the Translation of Impulse Into Action

Many factors besides impulsivity may influence the translation of impulse into action, including external circumstances and intoxication. Situational opportunities often modify the chances that an action will take place. This is well known to any clinician who asks a suicidal or paranoid patient if he or she has access to a firearm. Variations in suicide rates are due, in part, to differences in access to lethal methods of injury

(Marzuk et al. 1992). Use of drugs and alcohol can also promote impulsive behavior, because they interfere with the ability to integrate previous knowledge in the formulation of behavioral strategies (Lau and Pihl 1994).

Affective states influence the likelihood of action. Suicidal or aggressive impulses accompanied by strong affective states, such as depression or anger, are more likely to result in actual suicide or violence. These affective states magnify the intensity of the underlying impulse and diminish reflection. In one study, impulsive subjects who were depressed were more likely to be aggressive, but impulsive subjects who were not depressed were not more aggressive than nonimpulsive subjects (Hynan and Grush 1986). Thus, an impulse is more likely to result in aggression when it is emotionally triggered. Barratt (1993) has emphasized the role of strong emotional states or temper outbursts in impulsive aggression. He views impulsive aggression as a "hair-trigger response" in some people who do not process information in an adaptive way. Strong affect plays an important role in fostering risky or dangerous behavior in persons with borderline personality or bipolar disorders.

Social Aspects of Impulse Control: Socialization and Integration

Social and cultural forces play an important role in the development and maintenance of impulse control. Social standards often determine which impulses should be controlled. These standards have been incorporated into psychiatry's definitions of abnormal behaviors. Some unacceptable impulses are prominent in certain personality disorders and in impulse-control disorders.

There may be a split between standards of behavior imposed by society and the individual's own needs. More important, as these standards are internalized, a conflict arises within the person between moral imperatives and the need to gratify one's impulses. As a result of this internalization, the boundaries between social and psychological realms are blurred in humans. Prominent problems with impulse control can be indicative of some failure in socialization and may not be explained solely in biological terms.

Reconciling one's impulses to the demands of society is a fundamental developmental task that plays an important part in the formation of personality. A child acquires the cultural standards for the appropriate expression of various impulses; he or she must incorporate regulatory processes that allow automatic use of a large number of approved action patterns (Kluckhohn et al. 1953). As the child grows up, he or she learns to deal with various demands in increasingly more complex and flexible ways. Parents play a very important role in this socialization process; they have a direct impact on the child's acquisition of values through teaching and limit setting. In addition, through identification with parents, the child internalizes many of their values. When values and regulatory processes are fully integrated, they become an integral part of the person's sense of self (Deci et al. 1994).

The role of socialization should not be viewed solely in terms of inhibition and self-control. Solid values and rich personal relationships often exert an influence over a person's actions that makes active self-control unnecessary. Solid social bonds and awareness of social context enhance impulse regulation. Poor social integration, on the other hand, allows immediate demands—whether inner impulses or external exigencies—to control behavior. Impulse control requires that an individual become integrated within a family, a community, and a society—part of a system of human interactions in which there is "a constant interchange of ideas and feelings from all to each and each to all" (Durkheim 1951, p. 210).

It should be noted that the individual's ability to integrate socially is related to some of the very same biological factors as impulsivity. Serotonergic activity in nonhuman primates is negatively related to impulsivity or violence and positively related to sociality. Monkeys with higher concentrations of cerebrospinal fluid (CSF) 5-hydroxyindoleacetic acid (5-HIAA) perform better on various measures of affiliative sociality, including time spent grooming other monkeys, time in close proximity to others, and number of neighbors within a certain radius (Mehlman et al. 1995).

The individual's level of integration within society reflects to some extent the degree of social integration that exists in society as a whole. Durkheim (1951) believed that the propensity to attempt suicide in different societies reflects the degree of social disintegration within that society. This concept can be expanded to impulse control in general. Cohesive societies foster social integration that enables the individual to achieve better impulse control. Social disintegration, on the other hand, may reduce the threshold for impulsive behavior (Paris 1992).

The degree of control exerted over certain impulses depends in part on cultural norms. People may be much more inclined to certain behaviors, including violence, in cultures or subcultures where these are well tolerated or admired. It is important for clinicians to consider the overall adaptability of a behavior within a culture or subgroup before they consider it impulsive. In certain criminal groups, violence is instrumental to their occupations and not dysfunctional. These individuals can be contrasted to impulsive violent criminals, who have more unstable personality structures and less ability to function socially (Shoham et al. 1988).

Biological Aspects of Impulse Control

Overall Brain Structure and Impulse Control

Brain structure and function can provide a model for impulse control. Phylogenetically older brain structures can be viewed as the sites of instinctual drives or impulses of all sorts. These more primitive brain structures, which may be seen as a functional unit, are inhibited by newer cortical structures. Proper balance between these two functional systems is important for proper control of impulses. Inadequate impulse control can occur when there is hyperactivity of the more primitive brain structures, as occurs with stimulation or lesions of limbic areas, or inadequate control by the neocortex. In the latter case, impulses that are normally inhibited emerge spontaneously.

Moving up the phylogenetic scale from lower animals to human beings, we note considerable expansion of the newer cortical areas, especially the frontal lobes. This development enables humans to modulate their behavior more flexibly than animals can. We can integrate much more information, including social input, before we translate impulse into action. The cortical areas, and especially the frontal lobes, occupy a central role in impulse control, as well as in sociality, which is strongly related to impulse control. The mental structures underlying impulse control and sociality are not preprogrammed in the brain; they are developed in transactions with the environment. The ongoing interactions between biological and environmental factors provide an essential characteristic of human behavior: adaptability.

Release of inhibition can be chronic with certain lesions, tumors, or degenerative diseases. Lesions in frontal cortical areas, especially orbitofrontal areas, often result in prominent impulsivity (B. Kolb 1984). Impulsivity has also been reported with temporal lobe abnormalities, such as in patients with temporal lobe epilepsy (Herrington 1969) or patients with temporal lobe spiking on the electroencephalogram (EEG) (Treffert 1963). Temporal lobe epilepsy has to be considered in the differential diagnosis of impulse-control disorders such as pyromania, kleptomania, or intermittent explosive disorder (American Psychiatric Association 1994). Impulsivity can also be present with more generalized cortical impairment, as in Alzheimer's disease; disinhibited behaviors in that disorder increase with greater severity of dementia (Devanand et al. 1992).

Relationship Between Serotonin and Impulsivity

Although gross brain lesions underline the importance of certain brain areas in impulse control, they can provide only a limited view of much more complex and finely tuned mechanisms. Various neurotransmitter systems appear to be involved in impulse control. Subtle disruptions can occur in these systems without manifest neuronal destruction or degeneration. The relationship between one neurotransmitter, serotonin, and impulse control has received considerable attention in the literature over the past few years. In this section, this literature is selectively reviewed to evaluate some possible mechanisms of impulse control and to illustrate problems in understanding how biological variables influence behavior.

Animal Studies

Studies of serotonergic function were originally done in animals; the serotonergic system was seen as mediating different types of aggressive responses in a wide variety of species. More recently, elaborate information has been obtained on the intricate relationships between serotonin and aggression in nonhuman primates. Ratings of aggressivity in male rhesus monkeys were negatively related to CSF concentrations of 5-HIAA, the major serotonin metabolite (Higley et al. 1992a). Also in rhesus monkeys, low CSF 5-HIAA concentrations early in life predict later excessive risk taking, aggression, and premature death as a result of aggression (Higley et al. 1996). Beyond testing associations, researchers can experimentally manipulate serotonin levels. Decreasing serotonin in rats results in increased killing of mice (Eichelman and Thoa 1973; Gibbons et al. 1979), even in strains without a genetic predisposition to kill mice (Valzelli et al. 1981).

The animal work indicates that serotonin can influence several of the stages of the transformation of impulse into action. Serotonergic activity can modulate the strength of an impulse, or of an animal's sensitivity to stimuli, or facilitate a behavioral response. Depletion of serotonin results in a deficit in habituation to various stimuli (Conner et al.

1970). Increased rates of mouse killing in muricidal rats after a decrease in serotonergic activity may reflect an impairment in habituation. When rats have previously been exposed to mice, reduction of serotonergic activity has no effect on aggression (Marks et al. 1977; Vergnes and Kempf 1981). These rats had already become habituated, so the mice no longer constituted aversive stimuli.

Soubrie (1986) developed an animal model that he has applied to human impulsivity. In his model serotonin plays a general role in behavioral inhibition or the capacity to wait before action is undertaken. External factors—unfamiliar situations, punishment, or lack of reward—inhibit certain behaviors, which include aggression, exploration, and avoidance. Serotonin is involved in this inhibition or modulation of behavior. Decreased serotonin activity will result in "facilitation of responding"—that is, behavior will occur or persist even in the presence of external factors that are usually inhibitory (Whitaker-Azmitia et al. 1994). Soubrie (1986) termed this facilitation of behavioral response "impulsivity."

Some of the animal work illustrates that to understand the relationship between behavior and biological variables, such as serotonergic activity, it is necessary to consider the function of the behavior. Aggression can be just one of many means to serve a function; it may occur only when other behaviors are unsuitable or when there is inadequate opportunity to develop another response (File et al. 1979). When behavior is classified according to function, aggression is no longer a unitary concept; the same aggressive behavior can serve distinct functions, each with a different biological mechanism. Thus, in vervet monkeys, it is competitive aggression, but not spontaneous aggression, that is affected by decreases in serotonin levels (Chamberlain et al. 1987).

Human Studies

Serotonin and violence and suicide.   Most human studies of the role of serotonin in violence and suicide have investigated concentrations of serotonin metabolites, especially 5-HIAA, in the CSF. Other measures of serotonergic function—both peripheral (e.g., the tryptophan content in plasma or platelet serotonin uptake) and central (e.g., neuroendocrine challenges of central serotonin receptors, such as prolactin response after fenfluramine challenge)—have also been studied. Early investigators studied violence and suicide; the latter was often explained as a form of violence (i.e., self-directed violence). They found that serotonergic function was a marker and predictor of both violence and suicide.

An early, influential study found low levels of CSF 5-HIAA in depressive patients with histories of violent suicide attempts (Åsberg et al. 1976). In another pioneering study, lifetime aggression and suicide were associated with lower levels of CSF 5-HIAA in a group of 26 military men with various personality disorders and difficulties adjusting to military life (G. L. Brown et al. 1979). This finding was replicated in another study by the same group of researchers (G. L. Brown et al. 1982) involving 12 subjects with borderline personality disorder. Lifetime aggression and history of suicidal behavior were significantly associated with each other, and each was significantly associated with lower CSF levels of 5-HIAA. In a study comparing 15 murderers, 22 suicide attempters, and 39 control subjects (Lidberg et al. 1985), the suicidal patients, but not the murderers, had significantly lower CSF levels of 5-HIAA than the control subjects.

Serotonin and impulsive violence and suicide.   As additional studies were done, it became evident that serotonergic dysfunction was associated only with certain forms of violence or suicide, characterized as being either more severe or impulsive (G. L. Brown and Linnoila 1990; Mann 1987). (This distinction was also drawn in one study of nonhuman primates; in rhesus macaques only the more severe forms of aggression correlated with CSF levels of 5-HIAA, but the total rate of aggression did not [Mehlman et al. 1994].) The concept of impulsivity first emerged at this point in the development of the literature on biological aspects of human aggression. At this point the term *impulsive* was used to characterize the violence associated with low CSF levels of 5-HIAA. In one study, a group of impulsive offenders had lower mean CSF 5-HIAA concentrations than control subjects, but nonimpulsive offenders had higher concentrations than impulsive offenders and even the control subjects (Virkkunen et al. 1994).

The characterization of "impulsive violence," however, remained somewhat vague. Subjects were described as impulsive when their violence occurred "without provocation or premeditation" (Linnoila et al. 1983); this was judged to be so if the subject did not know the victim and investigators could detect no rationale for the aggression in psychiatric examination. In some studies of violent populations, impulsivity was explored as a dimension separate from violence; blood platelet uptake of serotonin (5-hydroxytryptamine) was negatively correlated with ratings of impulsivity as measured by the Barratt Impulsivity Scale in male outpatients with episodic aggression (C. S. Brown et al. 1989).

Serotonin and other impulsive behaviors.   Investigators have also studied other impulsive behavior, such as sexual disinhibition and arson, hypothesizing that low CSF levels of 5-HIAA reflect a disorder of poor impulse control rather than violence (Linnoila et al. 1989; Virkkunen et al. 1989). In one study, a group of 20 Finnish male arsonists had reduced CSF levels of 5-HIAA compared with habitually violent offenders and with control subjects. The authors believed that because arsonists are particularly impulsive but not violent, their results confirm the hypothesis that serotonergic function is associated primarily with poor impulse control rather than violence. Serotonin enhancement eliminates undesired sexual impulses and behaviors in human subjects (Zohar et al. 1994); it selectively reduces both paraphilias and nonparaphiliac sexual addictions (Kafka and Prentky 1992).

Possible environmental etiologies of serotonergic dysfunction. Environmental factors such as psychological trauma can affect both serotonergic function and impulsive behavior. Severe psychological trauma can result in persistent physiological disruptions, which include dysregulation of the serotonergic system (Higley et al. 1992b). Severe trauma may also have a disinhibitory effect on behavior (L. C. Kolb 1987). Traumatic experiences and social deprivation that occur early in life are particularly likely to permanently modify the serotonergic system (Kraemer and Clarke 1990). In monkeys, social separation in infancy results in changes in serotonin concentrations that persist into adulthood (Higley et al. 1991). These physiological disruptions may underlie the dysfunctional personality traits associated with severe psychological trauma, of which impulsivity is but one.

Substance abuse, particularly abuse of alcohol, can affect the serotonergic system. In studies that describe a serotonin deficit in impulsive, violent offenders and fire setters, all subjects were alcoholic individuals (Roy et al. 1987). Alcohol affects serotonin activity in many ways. It has a direct effect, depleting serotonin with chronic use. However, serotonergic depletion may be more pronounced during withdrawal and after 2 weeks of abstinence (Bailly et al. 1993). There is also evidence from animal studies that exposure to alcohol in utero decreases brain serotonin chronically and increases aggression (Krsiak et al. 1977). Studies that compare patients with a history of substance abuse with those without such a history have found that serotonergic dysfunction is specific to patients who abuse drugs or alcohol. In one such study (Moeller et al. 1994), there was a significant relationship between serotonergic dysfunction and aggression in cocaine-dependent patients but not in nondependent control subjects. Some of the studies reporting an association between serotonin deficit and impulsivity limited the subject population to patients with comorbid substance abuse disorder, such as patients with antisocial personality disorder with substance abuse (Moss et al. 1990). It is therefore important in future studies to provide information about subjects' substance abuse and to examine its contribution to serotonergic dysfunction.

However, the serotonergic dysfunction associated with alcoholism may not be environmentally determined. It can exist in the absence of actual alcohol intake, such as in nonalcoholic first-degree relatives of alcoholic individuals (Moss 1987), and may be indicative of a genetic predisposition to alcoholism. Even in alcoholic subjects, those with alcoholic fathers had a lower mean CSF 5-HIAA concentration than did those without alcoholic fathers (Linnoila et al. 1989). It is possible, then, to view alcoholism, itself, as part of a disinhibited behavioral pattern induced by serotonergic dysfunction (Bailly et al. 1993).

Global dysfunction and serotonergic abnormalities underlying impulsivity.   The distinction between functional and dysfunctional behaviors is very important when we interpret the impact of decreased serotonergic activity on behavior. The animal literature is primarily concerned with adaptive aggressive acts, whereas human studies focus on maladaptive behavior (Miczek et al. 1989). Therefore, extrapolations from animal neurophysiology to the human impairment associated with serotonergic dysfunction must be interpreted cautiously.

Human violent or impulsive behaviors appear to be part of a more generalized pattern of disturbed interpersonal relationships and abnormal behaviors. When impulsive behavior is studied in a group of psychiatrically healthy subjects, no relationship is found with serotonergic activity (af Klinteberg et al. 1992). Serotonergic dysfunction has been related to clinician and self-reported ratings of impulsive aggression only in patients with personality disorder, not in those with major affective disorder or in control subjects (Coccaro et al. 1989).

The criteria that investigators choose to characterize an action as impulsive may lead them to select as study subjects a group of more dysfunctional individuals in whom impulsivity is but one of many disturbances. For example, in several of the studies discussed earlier, "impulsive violence" was presumed to exist if the offender did not know the victim and had no discernible rationale for committing the act. Such criteria, however, not only may characterize impulsive violence but also suggest a generalized pattern of dysfunction in the offenders. People who have a history of chronic violence and suicide attempts, such as the subjects of several of the studies reviewed earlier, are likely to present with global difficulties that are reflected in a serious psychiatric disorder.

In the study of military personnel mentioned earlier (G. L. Brown et al. 1979), all of the impulsive and aggressive subjects had diagnoses of personality disorder; the disorder was so severe that the majority of these individuals were judged unsuitable for further military service. In another of the aforementioned studies (Linnoila et al. 1983), all subjects, whether they were impulsive or not, had some form of personality disorder, although the type and severity of the disorder differed markedly in the impulsive and nonimpulsive groups. The nonimpulsive criminals were given diagnoses of either paranoid or passive-aggressive personality disorders, diagnoses that presumably reflected the nature of their crimes. The impulsive criminals, on the other hand, presented with more severe disturbances. They all carried the diagnosis of borderline personality disorder, as well as intermittent explosive or antisocial personality disorder. Their pathology was of long duration, dating to childhood, when they presented with either attention-deficit/hyperactivity disorder or aggressive conduct disorder. Childhood disorders were rare in the nonimpulsive group.

In some studies both decreased serotonin concentration and impulsivity were found in certain dysfunctional individuals, but serotonergic activity was related to aggression or specific emotions, not impulsivity. It was negatively associated with assaultiveness and dysphoria but not with impulsivity in patients with antisocial personality disorder (Moss et al. 1990), and with aggression and expressed emotionality but not with impulsivity in children and adolescents with disruptive behavior disorders (Kruesi et al. 1990).

Impulsivity in the Context of Personality Disorder: Interplay Between Biological and Social Factors

Impulsivity is an important characteristic of both borderline and antisocial personality disorders. According to DSM-IV, impulsivity is evidenced in borderline personality disorder in potentially self-damaging acts such as drug abuse and recurrent suicidal gestures. In antisocial personality disorder, impulsivity manifests itself in a failure to plan ahead; decisions are made on the spur of the moment, without consideration for the consequences for self or others (American Psychiatric Association 1994).

In the context of personality disorders, impulsivity can be viewed as one facet of a more global dysfunction. In borderline personality disorder, it is part of a dysfunction in overall regulation of impulse, affect (Cowdry et al. 1991), and attachment or affiliation (M. West et al. 1993). Dysregulation in different spheres is interrelated; affective instability and chaotic interpersonal relationships can contribute to impulsive behavior.

The central feature of antisocial personality disorder is a pervasive pattern of disregard for the rights of others and irresponsibility (American Psychiatric Association 1994). Impulsivity is part of a lack of conventional social restraints (as manifested by, e.g., irregular work habits) and immoderation in the pursuit of immediate pleasure (e.g., through sexual activity or drug abuse) (D. J. West and Farrington 1973). Individuals with antisocial personality disorder appear to have shallow affect and insufficient capacity for attachment, as well as a general lack of empathy. Gottfredson and Hirschi (1990), in their description of the criminal offender, give a central role to lack of self-control over impulses and desires, in accordance with social restraints, as the main feature around which other traits are organized.

Impulsivity may emerge in these two disorders as a result of different transactions between biological predispositions and disruptions in the socialization process. Disturbances of the serotonergic system appear prominently in borderline personality disorder. Affective lability, impulsivity, and suicidal and aggressive behavior may all reflect serotonergic dysregulation. Traumatic disruptions in the developmental process, such as through physical or sexual abuse, often result in dysfunctional behavior patterns (Green 1978) and appear to play an important part in the formation of borderline pathology. Several studies have indicated greater prevalence of physical and sexual abuse in patients with borderline personality disorder (Goldman et al. 1992; J. B. Murray 1993). Certain authors (Gunderson and Sabo 1993; Westen et al. 1990) consider borderline psychopathology a consequence of a posttraumatic stress disorder. Such traumatic experiences, as described earlier, may result in permanent biological changes, including serotonergic dysfunction, and become incorporated in the personality structure.

Serotonergic abnormality does not seem as prevalent in antisocial personality disorder as in borderline personality disorder, especially when the antisocial acts are more functional. When present, it may reflect drug and alcohol abuse, which are common among persons with this disorder (Grande et al. 1984). Other dysfunctions may predispose to impulsive behavior in antisocial personality disorder, such as a low level of arousal and fear (Mednick and Moffit 1985).

Disturbances in socialization are of a different nature in antisocial compared with borderline personality disorder. Factors such as parental deviance or aggressiveness, parental conflict, and lack of parental supervision play an important role in the development of antisocial behavior (McCord 1979). The family or subculture may present a child with inadequate values—values at odds with the accepted societal norms—so that certain standards and regulatory inhibitory processes are not incorporated within the basic personality. This can become a powerful determinant of antisocial behavior when accompanied by certain biological propensities, such as a predisposition to fearlessness. Thus, impulsivity in antisocial personality disorder may be the result of a defective inhibition system with both biological and social etiologies. Behavior often remains adaptable and functional on a short-term basis, though a general disregard for others eventually has deleterious consequences.

Conclusion

In this chapter I reviewed biological, psychological, and social aspects of impulse control. The process of socialization emerged as a key concept. Society defines what constitutes unacceptable impulses; social structure influences the individual's impulse control. Because impulsive behaviors are discouraged in our society, their persistence into adulthood indicates a failure of socialization.

Serotonin appears to play an important role in social behaviors and sociality. It plays a central role in the "circuitry" of impulse control established through maturation of underlying brain structures in transactions with the environment. Reduced serotonin activity is associated with impaired impulse control. There are probably genetic predispositions for this decrease in serotonergic function, but environmental factors, such as early traumatic experiences or alcohol abuse, also play a role. Better understanding of these ongoing interactions or transactions will allow us to target our interventions to critical periods of development of certain children who have predispositions to impulsive and violent behaviors.

Impulse control cannot be understood without considering the function and adaptability of the behaviors elicited. For the most part, individuals will be able to adjust their behavior to meet societal norms, even in the presence of certain innate predispositions to impulsivity. Dysfunctional behavior is more likely to occur when there are major disruptions in the developmental process, such as when biological and social abnormalities interact in such a way as to affect the very adaptability of behavior, as occurs with antisocial and borderline personality disorders.

References

af Klinteberg B, Hallman J, Oreland L, et al: Exploring the connections between platelet monoamine oxidase activity and behavior, II: impulsive personality without neuropsychological signs of disinhibition in air force pilot recruits. Neuropsychobiology 26:136–145, 1992

American Psychiatric Association: Diagnostic and Statistical Manual of Mental Disorders, 4th Edition. Washington, DC, American Psychiatric Association, 1994

Åsberg M, Träskman L, Thorén P: 5-HIAA in the cerebrospinal fluid: a biochemical suicide predictor? Arch Gen Psychiatry 33:1193–1197, 1976

Bailly D, Vignau J, Racadot N, et al: Platelet serotonin levels in alcoholic patients: changes related to physiological and pathological factors. Psychiatry Res 47:57–88, 1993

Barratt ES: The use of anticonvulsants in aggression and violence. Psychopharmacol Bull 29:75–81, 1993

Brown CS, Kent TA, Bryant SG, et al: Blood platelet uptake of serotonin in episodic aggression. Psychiatry Res 27:5–12, 1989

Brown GL, Linnoila MI: CSF serotonin metabolite (5-HIAA) studies in depression, impulsivity, and violence. J Clin Psychiatry 51(no 4, suppl):31–41, 1990

Brown GL, Goodwin FK, Ballenger JC, et al: Aggression in humans correlates with cerebrospinal fluid amine metabolites. Psychiatry Res 1:131–139, 1979

Brown GL, Ebert MH, Goyer PF, et al: Aggression, suicide, and serotonin: relationships to CSF amine metabolites. Am J Psychiatry 139:741–746, 1982

Chamberlain B, Ervin FR, Pihl RO, et al: The effect of raising or lowering tryptophan levels on aggression in vervet monkeys. Pharmacol Biochem Behav 28:503–510, 1987

Coccaro EF, Siever LJ, Klar HM, et al: Serotonergic studies in patients with affective and personality disorders: correlates with suicidal and impulsive aggressive behavior. Arch Gen Psychiatry 46:587–599, 1989

Conner RL, Stolk JM, Barchas JD, et al: Parachlorophenylalanine and habituation to repetitive auditory startle stimuli in rats. Physiol Behav 5:1215–1219, 1970

Cowdry RW, Gardner DL, O'Leary KM, et al: Mood variability: a study of four groups. Am J Psychiatry 148:1505–1511, 1991

Deci EL, Eghrari H, Patrick BC, et al: Facilitating internalization: the self-determination theory perspective. J Pers 62:119–142, 1994

Devanand DP, Brockington CD, Moody BJ, et al: Behavioral syndromes in Alzheimer's disease. Int Psychogeriatr 4 (suppl 2):161–184, 1992

Durkheim E: Suicide: A Study in Sociology. Glencoe, IL, Free Press, 1951

Eichelman BS, Thoa NB: The aggressive monoamines. Biol Psychiatry 6:143–164, 1973

File SE, Hyde JR, MacLeod NK: 5,7-Dihydroxytryptamine lesions of dorsal and median raphe nuclei and performance in the social interaction test of anxiety and in a home-cage aggression test. J Affect Disord 1:115–122, 1979

Gibbons JL, Barr GA, Bridger WH, et al: Manipulations of dietary tryptophan: effects on mouse killing and brain serotonin in the rat. Brain Res 169:139–153, 1979

Goldman SJ, D'Angelo EJ, DeMaso DR, et al: Physical and sexual abuse histories among children with borderline personality disorder. Am J Psychiatry 149:1723–1726, 1992

Gottfredson MR, Hirschi TA: A General Theory of Crime. Stanford, CA, Stanford University Press, 1990

Grande TP, Wolf AW, Schubert DSP, et al: Associations among alcoholism, drug abuse, and antisocial personality: a review of the literature. Psychol Rep 55:455–474, 1984

Green AH: Self-destructive behavior in battered children. Am J Psychiatry 135:579–582, 1978

Gunderson JG, Sabo AN: The phenomenological and conceptual interface between borderline personality disorder and PTSD. Am J Psychiatry 150:19–27, 1993

Heilbrun AB: Psychopathy and violent crime. J Consult Clin Psychol 47:509–516, 1979

Herrington RN: The personality in temporal lobe epilepsy, in Current Problems in Neuropsychiatry (Br J Psychiatry Special Publ No 4).

Edited by Herrington RN. Ashford, Kent, UK, Headley Brothers, 1969

Higley JD, Suomi SJ, Linnoila M: CSF monoamine metabolite concentrations vary according to age, rearing, and sex, and are influenced by the stressor of social separation in rhesus monkeys. Psychopharmacology (Berl) 103:551–556, 1991

Higley JD, Mehlman PT, Taub DM, et al: Cerebrospinal fluid monoamine and adrenal correlates of aggression in free-ranging rhesus monkeys. Arch Gen Psychiatry 49:436–441, 1992a

Higley JD, Suomi SJ, Linnoila M: A longitudinal assessment of CSF monoamine metabolite and plasma cortisol concentrations in young rhesus monkeys. Biol Psychiatry 32:127–145, 1992b

Higley JD, Mehlman PT, Higley SB, et al: Excessive mortality in young free-ranging male nonhuman primates with low cerebrospinal fluid 5-hydroxyindoleacetic acid concentrations. Arch Gen Psychiatry 53:537–543, 1996

Hinsie L, Campbell RJ: Psychiatric Dictionary, 3rd Edition. New York, Oxford University Press, 1960

Hynan DJ, Grush JE: Effects of impulsivity, depression, provocation, and time on aggressive behavior. Journal of Research in Personality 20:158–171, 1986

Kafka MP, Prentky R: Fluoxetine treatment of nonparaphilic sexual addictions and paraphilias in men. J Clin Psychiatry 53:351–358, 1992

Kluckhohn C, Murray HA, Schneider D (eds): Personality in Nature, Society and Culture, 2nd Edition, New York, Knopf, 1953

Kolb B: Functions of the frontal cortex of the rat: a comparative review. Brain Res 320:65–98, 1984

Kolb LC: A neurophysiological hypothesis explaining posttraumatic stress disorders. Am J Psychiatry 144:989–995, 1987

Kraemer GW, Clarke AS: The behavioral neurobiology of self-injurious behavior in rhesus monkeys. Progr Neuropsychopharmacol Biol Psychiatry 14(suppl):S141–S168, 1990

Krsiak M, Elis J, Poschlova N, et al: Increased aggressiveness and lower brain serotonin levels in offspring of mice given alcohol during gestation. J Stud Alcohol 38:1696–1704, 1977

Kruesi MJ, Rapoport JL, Hamburger S, et al: Cerebrospinal fluid monoamine metabolites, aggression, and impulsivity in disruptive behavior disorders of children and adolescents. Arch Gen Psychiatry 47:419–426, 1990

Lau Ma, Pihl RO: Alcohol and the Taylor Aggression Paradigm: a repeated measures study. J Stud Alcohol 55:701–706, 1994

Lidberg L, Tuck JR, Åsberg M, et al: Homicide, suicide and CSF 5-HIAA. Acta Psychiatr Scand 71:230–236, 1985

Linnoila M, Virkkunen M, Scheinin M, et al: Low CSF 5-HIAA concentration differentiates impulsive from nonimpulsive violent behavior. Life Sci 33:2609–2614, 1983

Linnoila M, de Jong J, Virkkunen M: Family history of alcoholism in violent offenders and impulsive fire setters. Arch Gen Psychiatry 46:613–616, 1989

Mann JJ: Psychobiologic predictors of suicide. J Clin Psychiatry 48 (no 12, suppl):39–43, 1987

Marks PC, O'Brien M, Paxinos G: 5,7-DHT-induced muricide: inhibition as a result of preoperative exposure of rats to mice. Brain Res 135:383–388, 1977

Marzuk PM, Leon AC, Tardiff K, et al: The effect of access to lethal methods of injury on suicide rates. Arch Gen Psychiatry 49:451–458, 1992

McCord J: Some child-rearing antecedents of criminal behavior in adult men. J Pers Soc Psychol 37:1477–1486, 1979

Mednick SA, Moffit T (eds): Biology and Crime. Cambridge, UK, Cambridge University Press, 1985

Mehlman PT, Higley JD, Faucher I, et al: Low CSF concentrations and severe aggression and impaired impulse control in nonhuman primates. Am J Psychiatry 151:1485–1491, 1994

Mehlman PT, Higley JD, Faucher I, et al: Correlation of CSF 5-HIAA concentration with sociality and the timing of emigration in free-ranging primates. Am J Psychiatry 152:907–913, 1995

Miczek KA, Mos J, Olivier B: Brain 5-HT and inhibition of aggressive behavior in animals: 5-HIAA and receptor subtypes. Psychopharmacol Bull 25:399–403, 1989

Moeller FG, Steinberg JL, Petty F, et al: Serotonin and impulsive/aggressive behavior in cocaine dependent subjects. Progr Neuropsychopharmacol Biol Psychiatry 18:1027–1035, 1994

Moss HB: Serotonergic activity and disinhibitory psychopathy in alcoholism. Med Hypotheses 23:353–361, 1987

Moss HB, Yao JK, Panzak GL: Serotonergic responsivity and behavioral dimensions in antisocial personality disorder with substance abuse. Biol Psychiatry 28:325–338, 1990

Murray H: Explorations in Personality. New York, Oxford University Press, 1938

Murray JB: Relationship of childhood sexual abuse to borderline personality disorder, posttraumatic stress disorder, and multiple personality disorder. J Psychol 127:657–677, 1993

Paris J: Social risk factors for borderline personality disorder: a review and hypothesis. Can J Psychiatry 37:510–515, 1992

Roy A, Virkkunen M, Linnoila M: Reduced central serotonin turnover in a subgroup of alcoholics? Progr Neuropsychopharmacol Biol Psychiatry 11:173–177, 1987

Segal SP, Watson MA, Goldfinger SM, et al: Civil commitment in the psychiatric emergency room, III: disposition as a function of mental disorder and dangerousness indicators. Arch Gen Psychiatry 45:759–763, 1988

Shoham SG, Askenasy JJ, Rahav G, et al: Personality and social attitude correlates of violent prisoners. Med Law 7:269–286, 1988

Soubrie P: Reconciling the role of central serotonin neurons in human and animal behavior. Behav Brain Sci 9:319–363, 1986

Treffert DA: The psychiatric patient with an EEG temporal lobe focus. Am J Psychiatry 120:765–771, 1963

Valzelli L, Garattini S, Bernasconi S, et al: Neurochemical correlates of muricidal behavior in rats. Neuropsychobiology 7:172–178, 1981

Vergnes M, Kempf E: Tryptophan deprivation: effects on mouse-killing and reactivity in the rat. Pharmacol Biochem Behav 14 (suppl 1):19–23, 1981

Virkkunen M, Nuutila A, Goodwin FK, et al: Cerebrospinal fluid monoamine metabolite levels in male arsonists. Arch Gen Psychiatry 44:241–247, 1987

Virkkunen M, de Jong J, Barko J, et al: Relationship of psychobiological variables to recidivism in violent offenders and impulsive fire setters. Arch Gen Psychiatry 46:600–603, 1989

Virkkunen M, Rawlings R, Tokola R, et al: CSF biochemistries, glucose metabolism, and diurnal activity rhythms in alcoholic, violent offenders, fire setters, and healthy volunteers. Arch Gen Psychiatry 51:20–27, 1994

West DJ, Farrington DP: Who Becomes Delinquent? London, Heineman, 1973

West M, Keller A, Links P, et al: Borderline disorder and attachment pathology. Can J Psychiatry 38(suppl):S16–S22, 1993

Westen D, Ludolph P, Misle B, et al: Physical and sexual abuse in adolescent girls with borderline personality disorder. Am J Orthopsychiatry 60:55–66, 1990

Whitaker-Azmitia PM, Zhang X, Clarke C: Effects of gestational exposure to monoamine oxidase inhibitors in rats: preliminary behavioral and neurochemical studies. Neuropsychopharmacology 11:125–132, 1994

Zohar J, Kaplan Z, Benjamin J: Compulsive exhibitionism successfully treated with fluvoxamine: a controlled case study. J Clin Psychiatry 55:86–88, 1994

CHAPTER 9

Violence and Mental Disorder: Recent Research

John Monahan, Ph.D.

Nowhere is the change in contemporary understanding of the relationship between major mental disorder and violence more evident than in the public statements of groups advocating for people with mental disorder. Compare, for example, two statements issued in the late 1980s with two statements issued in the mid-1990s.

In 1987, the National Mental Health Association reiterated its oft-stated position that "people with mental illnesses pose no more of a crime threat than do other members of the general population" (p. 2). Shortly thereafter, the Well-Being Project (1989), a leading ex-patient advocacy group, stated that "studies show that while, like all groups, some members are violent, mental health clients are no more violent than the general population" (p. 88).

Several years later, however, the MacArthur Research Network on Mental Health and the Law collaborated with the National Stigma Clearinghouse, a family and consumer-oriented advocacy group, to produce a "Consensus Statement" that has been endorsed by a large number of researchers and advocates (Monahan and Arnold 1996). The statement frankly acknowledged that there is an association—albeit a weak one—between mental disorder and violence:

> "Mental disorder" and violence are closely linked in the public mind. A combination of factors promotes this perception: sensationalized reporting by the media whenever a violent act is committed by "a former mental patient," popular misuse of psychiatric terms (such as "psychotic" and "psychopathic"), and exploitation of stock formulas and narrow stereotypes by the entertainment industry. The public justifies its fear and rejection of people labeled "mentally ill," and attempts

to segregate them in the community, by this assumption of "danger-ousness."

The experience of people with psychiatric conditions and of their family members paints a picture dramatically different from the stereo-type. The results of several recent large-scale research projects conclude that only a weak association between mental disorders and violence exists in the community. Serious violence by people with major mental disorders appears concentrated in a small fraction of the total number, and especially in those who use alcohol and other drugs. Mental disor-ders—in sharp contrast to alcohol and drug abuse—account for a minuscule portion of the violence that afflicts American society.

The conclusions of those who use mental health services and of their family members, and the observations of researchers, suggest that the way to reduce whatever relationship exists between violence and mental disorder is to make accessible a range of quality treatments including peer-based programs, and to eliminate the stigma and discrimination that discourage, sometimes provoke, and penalize those who seek and receive help for disabling conditions. (Monahan and Arnold 1996, pp. 69–70)

Other advocates have recently come to the view that a relationship between mental disorder and violence should be not only acknowl-edged, as in the consensus statement, but also affirmatively *emphasized* by advocates for persons with mental disorder. For example, Jaffe (1994, p. 2), an official of the Alliance for the Mentally Ill, stated that "from a marketing perspective, it may be necessary to capitalize on the [public's] fear of violence to get the law passed" that would ensure that persons with mental disorder receive needed treatment (voluntarily or other-wise). For advocates to promote the potentially stigmatizing belief that persons with mental illness are prone to violence, he stated, "may be a bitter pill to swallow, but if it helps individuals with NBD [neurobiolog-ical disorders], I believe we should consider it" (Jaffe 1994, p. 2).

That advocates such as Jaffe would risk further stigmatizing persons with mental disorder as potentially violent is an indication of the lengths people will go to ensure that their loved ones receive treatment for mental disorder. Indeed, there is historical precedent for the effectiveness of fear-based arguments in securing resources for people with mental disorder.

The first general hospital in the American colonies to include a ward for people with mental disorders—the cellar—was founded at the urging of no less than Benjamin Franklin. After arguing in vain that the Penn-sylvania colony was morally obligated to provide for people with mental disorders, he switched tacks and petitioned the assembly in 1751 that "the Number of Persons distempered in Mind and deprived of their rational Faculties has increased greatly in this province. Some of them going at large are a terror to their Neighbors, who are daily apprehensive of the Violences they may commit" (quoted in Deutsch 1949, p. 59). This "provide treatment, or else" argument hit a responsive chord, and the Pennsylvania Hospital stands to this day in Philadelphia.

In this brief chapter I review four issues regarding the relationship between mental disorder and violent behavior, to put the claims of advocates into empirical context. Older studies have been reviewed by Mulvey (1994; see also Monahan 1992, 1996, 1997). I shall concentrate here, therefore, on work published since 1993. As a summary of prior work, I endorse Mulvey's conclusion that on the basis of the available literature, six statements could be made about the relationship between violence and mental disorder (Mulvey 1994, pp. 663–665):

1. Mental illness appears to be a risk factor for violence in the community. A body of research, taken as a whole, supports the idea that an association exists between mental illness and violence in the general population.
2. The size of the association between mental illness and violence, while statistically significant, does not appear to be very large. Also, the absolute risk for violence posed by mental illness is small.
3. The combination of a serious mental illness and a substance abuse disorder probably significantly increases the risk of involvement in a violent act.
4. The association between mental illness and violence is probably significant even when demographic characteristics are taken into account. However, no sizeable body of evidence clearly indicates the relative strength of mental illness as a risk factor for violence compared with other characteristics such as socioeconomic status or history of violence.
5. Active symptoms are probably more important as a risk factor than is simply the presence of an identifiable disorder.
6. No clear information about the causal paths that produce the association between mental illness and violence is available.

As Wessely et al. (1994) have stated:

Viewed in terms of attributable risk, the contribution made by those with schizophrenia to the level of recorded crime in the community is slender. The strongest predictors of crime in those with schizophrenia are the same as those in subjects without psychosis. Nevertheless, serious mental illness also exerts a small, but significant independent effect on recorded crime. Low risk is not the same as no risk, and these findings must be taken seriously. (p. 500)

Issue One: Symptoms and Violence

Link and Stueve (1994) reanalyzed the data used in a study by Link et al. (1992) to allow for a much more precise specification of *what kind* of "psychotic symptoms" are most related to violence. They found that three symptoms on the psychotic symptoms scale largely explained the relationship between mental disorder and violence.[1] The authors referred to these as "threat/control-override symptoms," because they either involve the overriding of internal self-controls by external factors (items 1 and 2) or imply a specific threat of harm from others (item 3). Link and Stueve (1994, p. 143) explained their results by invoking a principle of "rationality-within-irrationality":

> The principle of rationality-within-irrationality posits that once one suspends concern about the irrationality of psychotic symptoms and accepts that they are experienced as real, violence unfolds in a "rational" fashion. By rational we do not mean reasonable or justified but rather understandable. Specifically, we suggest that when a person fears personal harm or feels threatened by others[,] interpersonal violence becomes more likely. In addition we argue that violence is more likely when internal controls that might otherwise block the expression of violence break down. From this perspective the nature and content of the psychotic experience become important. If the psychotic experience involves the removal of self-control through, for example, thought insertion or having one's mind dominated by outside forces, routine, self-imposed constraints on behavior are more likely to be overridden, and violence becomes a greater possibility. Further, if the afflicted person believes that he or she is gravely threatened by someone who intends to cause harm, violence is again more likely. In contrast, if the psychotic episode involves odd experiences such as hearing voices, seeing visions, or having one's thoughts taken away, without the intrusion of external, uncontrollable, and threatening forces, violence is less likely.

Swanson et al. (1996) replicated Link and Stueve's (1994) central finding with data from the Epidemiologic Catchment Area (ECA) study. They found that respondents who reported threat/control-override symptoms were twice as likely as those with other psychotic symptoms, and about six times as likely as those with no mental disorder, to report

---

[1] The items were "During the past year . . . (1) 'How often have you felt that your mind was dominated by forces beyond your control?'; (2) 'How often have you felt that thoughts were put into your head that were not your own?'; and (3) 'How often have you felt that there were people who wished to do you harm?'"

violence. People with threat/control-override symptoms combined with alcohol or other drug use disorders were 8–10 times more likely to report violence than those without mental disorder.

Link et al. (1999) again replicated the relationship between threat/control-override symptoms and violence, this time among a large epidemiological sample of the general population of Israel. However, Appelbaum et al. (in press) failed to find any effect for threat/control-override symptoms in the MacArthur Violence Risk Assessment Study.

Issue Two: Accuracy of Clinical Predictions of Violence

Lidz et al. (1993), in what is surely the most sophisticated study published on the clinical prediction of violence, took as their subjects male and female patients being examined in the acute psychiatric emergency room of a large civil hospital. Psychiatrists and nurses were asked to assess potential patient violence to others over the next 6-month period. Violence was measured by official records, by patient self-report, and by the report of a collateral informant in the community (e.g., a family member). Patients who elicited professional concern regarding future violence were found to be significantly more likely to be violent after release (53%) than were patients who had not elicited such concern (36%). The accuracy of clinical prediction did not vary as a function of the patient's age or race. The accuracy of clinicians' predictions of violence among male patients substantially exceeded chance levels for patients with and without a prior history of violent behavior. In contrast, the accuracy of clinicians' predictions of violence among female patients did not differ from chance. Although the actual rate of violent incidents among released female patients (46%) was higher than the rate among released male patients (42%), the clinicians had predicted that only 22% of the women, compared with 45% of the men, would be violent. (For research on the communication of risk assessments such as these, see Slovic and Monahan 1995 and Monahan and Steadman 1996.)

Issue Three: Accuracy of Actuarial Predictions of Violence

Borum (1996) has reminded us that a wide range of instruments can be subsumed under the rubric of "actuarial" prediction:

> At a minimum, these devices can serve as a checklist for clinicians to
> ensure that essential areas of inquiry are recalled and evaluated. At
> best, they may be able to provide hard actuarial data on the probability
> of violence among people (and environments) with a given set of char-
> acteristics, circumstances, or both. (p. 948)

A major advance in the development of actuarial risk assessment
was reported by Harris et al. (1993) (see also Rice 1997). A sample of 618
men who were either treated or administered a pretrial assessment at a
maximum-security forensic hospital in Canada served as subjects. All
had been charged with a serious criminal offense. A wide variety of
predictive variables were coded from institutional files.[2] The criterion
variable was any new criminal charge for a violent offense, or return to
the institution for an act that would otherwise have resulted in such a
charge. The average follow-up period was almost 7 years.

Results from multiple discriminant analyses indicated that the actuarial instrument yielded a multiple R of 0.46 with violent recidivism.
Classification accuracy was approximately 75%. Harris et al. (1993)
concluded:

> Clinical judgment can be improved . . . through the use of actuarial
> information; this has been referred to as "structuring discretion." In
> this approach to decision making about an individual, an actuarial esti-
> mate of risk is used to anchor clinical judgment. More specifically, clini-
> cians can use dynamic (changeable) information such as progress in
> treatment, change in procriminal attitudes, and the amount and quality
> of supervision in the postrelease environment to adjust the risk level
> computed by the actuarial prediction instrument. If adjustments are
> made conservatively and *only* when a clinician believes, on good
> evidence, that a factor is related to the likelihood of violent recidivism
> in an individual case, predictive accuracy may be improved. (p. 331)

As the authors noted, additional research is necessary to determine
the degree to which the impressive validity of these actuarial predictions
can be generalized to other populations. Attempts at cross-validating

---

[2] Twelve variables were identified for inclusion in the final statistical prediction instrument. The variables were a) score on the Hare Psychopathy Checklist—Revised, b) separation from parents under age 16, c) victim injury in index offense, d) DSM-III schizophrenia, e) never married, f) elementary school maladjustment, g) female victim in index
offense, h) failure on prior conditional release, i) property offense history, j) age at index
offense, k) alcohol abuse history, and l) DSM-III personality disorder. For all variables,
except c, d, g, and j, the nature of the relationship to subsequent violence was positive.
(That is, subjects who injured a victim in the index offense, who were diagnosed as having
schizophrenia, who chose a female victim for the index offense, or who were older were
significantly *less* likely to be violent recidivists than were other subjects.)

other instruments have yielded problematic results (Klassen and O'Connor 1990).

Gardner et al. (1996) recently have made an important methodological contribution to the use of actuarial information in predicting violence by civil patients in the community. They contrasted the usual "regression equation" model—in which points for various risk factors are summed to yield a prediction score, to which cutoffs are applied—with newer "regression tree" methods.

> A regression tree is a structured sequence of yes/no questions that lead to the classification of a case. . . . Statistical predictions requiring calculations may be infeasible in many clinical settings, while a decision procedure specified by a tree is easy to perform. A regression tree is also easy to grasp and explain because it generates a series of statements about a patient that provide reasons for the prediction. We therefore believe that clinicians will be more likely to accept regression trees than numerical formulas as methods for making actuarial predictions. (pp. 36–37)

The four yes/no questions contained in the Gardner et al. (1996) regression tree were "Is BSI Hostility greater than 2?" (i.e., is the patient's score on the Hostility subscale of the Brief Symptom Inventory [Derogatis and Melisaratos 1983] greater than 2?), "Is age less than 18?," "Is the patient a heavy drug user?," and "Are there more than three prior violent acts?" When applied to the data set used by Lidz et al. (1993), described earlier in this chapter, this regression tree identified a small group of patients (3% of the patient population) who committed violent acts at the high rate of 2.75 incidents per month (see also Monahan 1997).

More information on risk factors that actuarially relate to violence among populations of persons with mental disorder is available from the MacArthur Risk Assessment Study (Steadman et al. 1994). This research assessed a large sample of male and female acute civil patients at several facilities on a wide variety of variables believed to be related to the occurrence of violence. The risk factors fall into four domains. One domain consists of "dispositional" variables, which refer to, for example, the demographic factors of age, race, gender, and social class, as well as to personality variables (e.g., impulsivity and anger control) and neurological factors (e.g., head injury). A second domain consists of "historical" variables, which include significant events experienced by subjects in the past, such as family history, work history, mental hospitalization history, history of violence, and criminal and juvenile justice history. A third domain consists of "contextual" variables, which refer to indices of current social supports, social networks, and stress, as well as to physical aspects of the environment, such as the presence of weapons. The final domain consists of "clinical" variables, which include types and symptoms of mental disorder, personality disorder, drug and alcohol abuse, and level of functioning. The study is investigating the association between variables from each of these four domains and violence occurring in the community. Community violence is measured during interviews with the patients and with a collateral that occur five times over the course of a 1-year postrelease follow-up, as well as from official records. Complete results from this study are only now being published (Monahan et al., in press; Steadman et al. 1998, in press).

Issue Four: Implications for Law and Policy

Do any implications for law and public policy flow from the conclusions that persons with acute mental disorder have a modestly elevated risk of violence and that clinicians have modest abilities to predict this violence? Five controversial implications have in fact already been drawn from these studies by E. Fuller Torrey (1994), a well-known psychiatrist, and by D. J. Jaffe (1994), a board member of the Alliance for the Mentally Ill who was cited earlier.

1. *Substantive standards for involuntary commitment should be broadened.* "Danger to self or others" as the legal standard for involuntary commitment should be supplemented, according to Jaffe (1994, p. 2), by "need for treatment" (for persons "who are unable to comprehend the treatment being proposed or its likely courses and outcomes") and "grave disability" (for persons who "have deteriorated to the point where they are no longer able to provide for their own welfare"). The addition of such standards would allow involuntary intervention to take place "before the individual becomes a danger to self or others, thus avoiding needless violence and another stigmatizing headline."

2. *Evidentiary criteria for involuntary commitment should be loosened.* Torrey (1994) states that in many jurisdictions evidence of "dangerousness to others" in commitment statutes is limited to acts occurring in the previous 30 days. Such statutes should be broadened to allow evidence bearing on "the most important predictors of dangerousness, such as medication noncompliance, history of violent behavior [regardless of whether the noncompliance or violence occurred within the past 30 days], and concurrent drug and alcohol abuse" (p. 660).

3. *Committed patients should not be accorded a right to refuse medication.* For the law to permit involuntary commitment without involuntary treatment "makes no sense" to Torrey (1994, p. 660) and is "a ludicrous proposition" to Jaffe (1994, p. 2).

4. *The use of (prehospital) outpatient commitment should be expanded.* Outpatient commitment laws mandating medication or other treatments are in effect in most states but are not widely used. They should be, according to Jaffe (1994, p. 2), because the use of outpatient commitment "would cut down on the number of people who deteriorate to dangerousness because they have stopped treatment."

5. *The use of (posthospital) outpatient commitment should be expanded.* The release of persons with serious mental illness and a history of violence from mental hospitals should be made conditional upon their remaining in supervised aftercare. (The same proposal is made for persons with serious mental disorder and a history of violence being released from jails and prisons as well, but this raises different issues). The conditional release and mandatory community monitoring provisions used for forensic patients are recommended by Torrey (1994) as a model for civil patients as well.

Many patient advocates strongly contest these implications drawn by Torrey and Jaffe. Whatever their ultimate impact on mental health law may be, however, the findings reported in the more recent studies of mental disorder and violence reviewed in this chapter may have clear implications for mental health *practice.* For example, if the base rates of violence among persons with certain types of acute mental disorder are indeed somewhat higher than among persons without such disorder, and if among people with certain types of mental disorder given symptom patterns are associated with a disproportionate likelihood of violence, clinical training, and ultimately day-to-day clinical practice, should reflect these results. As Steadman et al. (1994) stated,

> [If ongoing research] is successful in its efforts to establish robust markers of violence risk, future research might address optimum methods of educating clinicians in the use of these markers. In that manner, the validity of clinical risk management could be appreciably improved. (p. 316)

References

Appelbaum P, Robbins P, Monahan J: Violence and delusions: data from the MacArthur Violence Risk Assessment Study. Am J Psychiatry (in press)

Borum R: Improving the clinical practice of violence risk assessment: technology, guidelines, and training. Am Psychol 51:945–956, 1996

Derogatis L, Melisaratos N: The Brief Symptom Inventory: an introductory report. Psychol Med 13:595–605, 1983

Deutsch A: The Mentally Ill in America: A History of Their Care and Treatment From Colonial Times, 2nd Edition. New York, Columbia University Press, 1949

Gardner W, Lidz C, Mulvey E, et al: A comparison of actuarial methods for identifying repetitively violent patients with mental illness. Law and Human Behavior 20:35–48, 1996

Harris G, Rice M, Quinsey V: Violent recidivism of mentally disordered offenders: the development of a statistical prediction instrument. Criminal Justice and Behavior 20:315–335, 1993

Jaffe DJ: How to reduce both violence and stigma. Innovations and Research 3:1–2, 1994

Klassen D, O'Connor W: Assessing the risk of violence in released mental patients: a cross-validation study. Psychological Assessment: A Journal of Consulting and Clinical Psychology 1:75–81, 1990

Lidz C, Mulvey E, Gardner W: The accuracy of predictions of violence to others. JAMA 269:1007–1011, 1993

Link B, Stueve A: Psychotic symptoms and the violent/illegal behavior of mental patients compared to community controls, in Violence and Mental Disorder: Developments in Risk Assessment. Edited by Monahan J, Steadman H. Chicago, IL, University of Chicago Press, 1994, pp 137–159

Link B, Andrews H, Cullen F: The violent and illegal behavior of mental patients reconsidered. American Sociological Review 57:275–292, 1992

Link B, Monahan J, Stueve A, et al: Real in their consequences: a sociological approach to understanding the association between psychotic symptoms and violence. American Sociological Review 64:316–332, 1999

Monahan J: Mental disorder and violent behavior: perceptions and evidence. Am Psychol 47:511–521, 1992

Monahan J: Violence prediction: the last twenty and the next twenty years. Criminal Justice and Behavior 23:107–120, 1996

Monahan J: Clinical and actuarial predictions of violence, in Modern Scientific Evidence: The Law and Science of Expert Testimony. Edited by Faigman D, Kaye D, Saks M, et al. St Paul, MN, West Publishing Company, 1997, pp 300–318

Monahan J: Actuarial support for the clinical assessment of violence risk. International Review of Psychiatry 9:167–169, 1997

Monahan J, Arnold J: Violence by people with mental illness: a consensus statement by advocates and researchers. Psychiatric Rehabilitation Journal 19:67–70, 1996

Monahan J, Steadman H: Violent storms and violent people: how meteorology can inform risk communication in mental health law. Am Psychol 51:931–938, 1996

Monahan J, Steadman H, Appelbaum P, et al: Developing a clinically useful actuarial tool for assessing violence risk. Br J Psychiatry (in press)

Mulvey E: Assessing the evidence of a link between mental illness and violence. Hospital and Community Psychiatry 45:663–668, 1994

National Mental Health Association: Stigma: A Lack of Awareness and Understanding. Alexandria, VA, National Mental Health Association, 1987

Rice M: Violent offender research and implications for the criminal justice system. Am Psychol 52:414–423, 1997

Slovic P, Monahan J: Danger and coercion: a study of risk perception and decision making in mental health law. Law and Human Behavior 19:49–65, 1995

Steadman H, Monahan J, Appelbaum P, et al: Designing a new generation of risk assessment research, in Violence and Mental Disorder: Developments in Risk Assessment. Edited by Monahan J, Steadman H. Chicago, IL, University of Chicago Press, 1994, pp 297–318

Steadman H, Mulvey E, Monahan J, et al: Violence by people discharged from acute psychiatric inpatient facilities and by others in the same neighborhoods. Arch Gen Psychiatry 55:393–401, 1998

Steadman H, Silver E, Monahan J, et al: A classification tree approach to the development of actuarial violence risk assessment tools. Law and Human Behavior (in press)

Swanson J, Borum R, Swartz M, et al: Psychotic symptoms and disorders and the risk of violent behaviour in the community. Criminal Behaviour and Mental Health 6:317–338, 1996

Torrey E: Violent behavior by individuals with serious mental illness. Hospital and Community Psychiatry 45:653–662, 1994

Well-Being Project: The Well-Being Project: Mental Health Clients Speak for Themselves. Sacramento, California Department of Mental Health, 1989

Wessely S, Castle D, Douglas A, et al: The criminal careers of incident cases of schizophrenia. Psychol Med 24:483–502, 1994

Index

*Page numbers printed in **boldface** type refer to tables or figures.*